FACIAL
ENHANCEMENT
ACUPUNCTURE

of related interest

Japanese Holistic Face Massage
Rosemary Patten
ISBN 978 1 84819 122 8
eISBN 978 0 85701 100 8

Vital Face
Facial Exercises and Massage for Health and Beauty
Leena Kiviluoma
ISBN 978 1 84819 166 2
eISBN 978 0 85701 130 5

Acupuncture for New Practitioners
John Hamwee
ISBN 978 1 84819 102 0
eISBN 978 0 85701 083 4

FACIAL ENHANCEMENT ACUPUNCTURE

Clinical Use and Application

PAUL ADKINS

PHOTOGRAPHS BY ROGER DUTTON

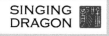

SINGING DRAGON

Figures 1.1 and 3.1–3.7 have been purchased and adapted from
iStockphoto.com in accordance with their Standard Licence.
Figure 1.1 © iStockphoto.com/LindaMarieB.
Figures 3.1–3.6 © iStockphoto.com/ariwasabi.
Figure 3.7 © iStockphoto.com/Gangliulo.
Figures 4.1–5.14 are reproduced with kind permission from Roger Dutton.
All photographs have been edited and enhanced by Stacey George.

First published in 2014
by Singing Dragon
an imprint of Jessica Kingsley Publishers
73 Collier Street
London N1 9BE, UK
and
400 Market Street, Suite 400
Philadelphia, PA 19106, USA

www.singingdragon.com

Copyright © Paul Adkins 2014
Photography copyright © Roger Dutton 2014

Front cover image source: Shutterstock®. The cover image is for
illustrative purposes only, and any person featuring is a model.

Library of Congress Cataloging in Publication Data
A CIP catalog record for this book is available from the Library of Congress

British Library Cataloguing in Publication Data
A CIP catalogue record for this book is available from the British Library

ISBN 978 1 84819 129 7
eISBN 978 0 85701 103 9

Printed and bound in China

CONTENTS

DISCLAIMER   9

ACKNOWLEDGEMENTS   10

PREFACE   11

1   INTRODUCTION TO FACIAL ENHANCEMENT ACUPUNCTURE   13
1.1   The Five Elements   13
1.1.1 The Wood Element   15
1.1.2 The Officials of the Wood Element   17
1.1.3 The Wood Element Facial Patient   20
1.1.4 The Fire Element   20
1.1.5 The Officials of the Fire Element   21
1.1.6 The Fire Element Facial Patient   24
1.1.7 The Earth Element   24
1.1.8 The Officials of the Earth Element   26
1.1.9 The Earth Element Facial Patient   28
1.1.10 The Metal Element   28
1.1.11 The Officials of the Metal Element   30
1.1.12 The Metal Element Facial Patient   32
1.1.13 The Water Element   33
1.1.14 The Officials of the Water Element   35
1.1.15 The Water Element Facial Patient   36
1.2   The History of Facial Acupuncture   37
1.3   Modern-Day Treatment Comparison   39
1.4   The Development of Facial Enhancement Acupuncture   41
1.4.1 The Muscles of the Face   42
1.4.2 Lines and Wrinkles   44

2   EXPECTED RESULTS OF FACIAL ENHANCEMENT
    ACUPUNCTURE   46

3   ACUPUNCTURE POINTS USED IN THE MAIN PROTOCOL   50
3.1   The Aggressive Energy Treatment (AE Drain)   50
3.2   Acupuncture Points on the Feet and Legs   51
3.3   Acupuncture Points on the Hands and Arms   54
3.4   Acupuncture Points on the Head and Forehead   58
3.5   Acupuncture Points around the Eyes   62
3.6   Acupuncture Points on the Jaw   65
3.7   Acupuncture Points on the Front of the Face   66
3.8   Acupuncture Point on the Chin   70
3.9   Acupuncture Points to Treat the Neck   71
3.10   Auricular Acupuncture Points for Facial Enhancement Acupuncture   76

**4   STEP-BY-STEP GUIDE TO THE FACIAL ENHANCEMENT
      ACUPUNCTURE PROTOCOL   82**

4.1   Contraindications   82
4.2   Preparation   83
4.3   Step-by-Step Guide to Facial Enhancement Acupuncture   83
4.3.1 Initial Grounding Treatment   83
4.3.2 Needling the Legs and Feet   85
4.3.3 Needling the Hands and Arms   85
4.3.4 Needling the Head and Forehead   85
4.3.5 Needling the Ears   91
4.3.6 Needling the Eyebrow Area   92
4.3.7 Needling the Jaw   94
4.3.8 Needling the Front of the Face   96
4.3.9 Needling the Chin 102
4.3.10 Treating the Neck 103
4.3.11 Treating Wrinkles 106
4.3.12 Applying Serums and Creams 116
4.4   Facial Enhancement Acupressure Massage 118
4.4.1 Massage Stage 1 120
4.4.2 Massage Stage 2 123
4.4.3 Massage Stage 3 124
4.4.4 Massage Stage 4 126
4.4.5 Massage Stage 5 127
4.4.6 Massage Stage 6 130
4.5   Finishing the Treatment 132

5   ADVANCED FACIAL ENHANCEMENT TECHNIQUES   133

5.1   Jade Gua Sha 133
5.1.1 About Gua Sha 133
5.1.2 The Gua Sha Facial Massage 135
5.2   Jade Rollers 138
5.2.1 About Jade Rollers 138
5.2.2 Step-by-Step Jade Roller Facial Massage 139
5.3   Dermal Rollers 150
5.3.1 About Dermal Rollers 150
5.3.2 How Skin Needling Works 150

6   TREATING SPECIFIC FACIAL ISSUES   154

6.1   The Acupuncture Meridians and their Role in Facial Enhancement Acupuncture . . 154
6.2   Sagging Facial Muscles 157
6.3   Eye Bags and Dark Circles 157
6.4   Age Spots and Skin Discolouration 159
6.5   Acne 159
6.6   Eczema 160
6.7   Rosacea 161

7   FACIAL ENHANCEMENT ACUPUNCTURE CASE STUDIES   163

7.1   Case Study 1: Jane, Aged 58 163
7.2   Case Study 2: Petra, Aged 35 165
7.3   Sample Case Studies 167

8.1   **Marketing to Existing Patients** 176
8.2   **Attracting New Patients** 178
8.3   **Online Marketing** 180
8.4   **Memberships** 182
8.5   **Branding** 183
8.6   **Top Ten Marketing Tips for Facial Enhancement Acupuncture** 183

GLOSSARY   185

RESOURCES   187

REFERENCES   189

LIST OF FIGURES

Figure 1.1   The face and neck muscles 44
Figure 3.1   The location of the head and forehead points. 62
Figure 3.2   The location of the points used around the eyes 64
Figure 3.3   The positioning of the jaw points. 65
Figure 3.4   The location of the points used on the front of the face 69
Figure 3.5   The location of Ren 24. 71
Figure 3.6   The location of the points used on the neck 76
Figure 3.7   The location of the auricular points 1–18 78
Figure 4.1   Demonstrating needling at Yin Tang. 87
Figure 4.2   Demonstrating needling in the hairline at BL6. 88
Figure 4.3   Demonstrating needling at GB14 89
Figure 4.4   Demonstrating needling at the Extra forehead point 90
Figure 4.5   Demonstrating needling at the auricular point Shen Men 91
Figure 4.6   Demonstrating needling at Yuyao and the intradermal needling technique
               using wide grip tweezers 92
Figure 4.7   Demonstrating the eyebrow needles in place 93
Figure 4.8   Locating the first jaw point and tucking the skin beneath the jaw bone 95
Figure 4.9   Demonstrating needling along the jaw line. 95
Figure 4.10   Demonstrating how to needle the Extra cheek point 96
Figure 4.11   Demonstrating needling at ST4 97
Figure 4.12   Demonstrating needling at LI20 98
Figure 4.13   Demonstrating needling at ST3 99
Figure 4.14   Demonstrating needling at SI18 100
Figure 4.15   Demonstrating needling at ST2 101
Figure 4.16   Demonstrating needling at Ren 24. 103
Figure 4.17   Demonstrating needling at SI17 103
Figure 4.18   Demonstrating needling at Ren 23. 105
Figure 4.19   Demonstrating needling at ST9 105
Figure 4.20   Demonstrating intradermal needling at the 'number elevens'. 109
Figure 4.21   A close-up of intradermal needling in a forehead line. 111
Figure 4.22   Demonstrating intradermal needling in the forehead lines 111
Figure 4.23   Demonstrating the intradermal needling technique at the base of
               the nasal labial fold. 113
Figure 4.24   Demonstrating intradermal needling along the nasal labial fold 113
Figure 4.25   Demonstrating intradermal needling on the 'crow's feet' 114

Figure 4.26   Demonstrating intradermal needling along the top lip, chin and
               the bridge of the nose 115
Figure 4.27   Placing thumbs above Yin Tang to begin the facial massage 121
Figure 4.28   Sliding both thumbs across the forehead 121
Figure 4.29   Using a circular motion at the temple 122
Figure 4.30   Using the middle fingers to massage the forehead with continuous strokes . . . 123
Figure 4.31   Begin by placing your thumbs at LI20 125
Figure 4.32   Sweep down the nasal labial fold 125
Figure 4.33   Applying pressure to point ST4 126
Figure 4.34   Continuously stroking the chin in an upwards direction using each thumb . . 127
Figure 4.35   Begin with thumbs placed at ST9 128
Figure 4.36   Gently sweeping the thumbs up the neck 129
Figure 4.37   Finishing the stroke from ST9 beneath the ears 129
Figure 4.38   Holding the tension on the cheeks up towards the ears. 130
Figure 4.39   Placing both hands, with fingers touching at the centre of the neck 131
Figure 4.40   Sweeping upward strokes on the neck area 131
Figure 5.1   Using gentle pressure to sweep the jade Gua Sha stone
               from the neck to the ear 135
Figure 5.2   Working on the nasal labial fold 136
Figure 5.3   Massaging the forehead lines with the tip of the Gua Sha stone 137
Figure 5.4   Rolling the jade roller from the ear to the mouth. 139
Figure 5.5   Moving the jade roller across to focus on the nasal labial fold 140
Figure 5.6   Using the large jade roller to massage the neck 141
Figure 5.7   Rolling the large jade roller up and down the side of the eye 143
Figure 5.8   Turning the large jade roller 90 degrees to roll up to the eye 143
Figure 5.9   Sweeping the large jade roller across the face 144
Figure 5.10   Using the small jade roller to roll across the nasal labial fold 145
Figure 5.11   The small jade roller is used on the chin area. 146
Figure 5.12   Targeting the top lip area with the small jade roller. 147
Figure 5.13   Rolling the 'crow's feet' with the small jade roller. 148
Figure 5.14   Using the small jade roller to smooth the 'number elevens'. 149

DISCLAIMER

The techniques and methods described in this publication are based on the author's knowledge and personal experience and no guarantees can be made as to their accuracy or success. The author can take no responsibility whatsoever for the results of any treatment that someone decides to carry out after reading this publication. In no circumstances should the information contained in this book be used as a guide for medical practice or purpose. If a medical condition is suspected, then you are advised to consult a medical practitioner, particularly if you are on orthodox medication.

ACKNOWLEDGEMENTS

This book has been made possible by the love, support and encouragement of so many people.

First, I want to acknowledge the help and support of my partner Stacey George. Without her editorial assistance, design work and expertise in research, this book would not have come together on time, if at all. She is an accomplished Feng Shui practitioner and Chinese astrologist and I am sure has many of her own books to write.

Also, I would like to thank Julie George for her role as our model for the Step-by-Step Guide. Her patience was greatly appreciated. These photographs were all taken by a very good friend, Roger Dutton. His dedication and skill with the camera is second to none.

I would also like to extend thanks to my three great children who I am so proud of, and my fantastic parents who have always been there for me and encouraged me to set my sights high.

I would like to acknowledge and thank all of the staff and my fellow students who attended the College of Traditional Acupuncture in Leamington Spa, England. I have been honoured to have been taught by some of the finest minds in Five Element Acupuncture and without their support and encouragement I would not be publishing this book today.

My appreciation goes to my demonstration patients and the students who undertake my courses. You continue to inspire me with your enthusiasm for Facial Enhancement Acupuncture, which vastly helps the continual progression of the protocol.

My thanks go to Jessica Kingsley Publishers for their faith in me and their help with this publication.

Thank you, everyone, for your assistance, and I hope this book justifies your support.

PREFACE

I first started my journey into acupuncture in the year 2000 at the age of 40, quite late compared to many other practitioners. My entire working life was previously involved in sales and marketing, of one type or another, so studying acupuncture was a whole new departure for me.

I studied Classical Five Element Acupuncture at the CTA College of Traditional Acupuncture in Leamington Spa, England, and gained an honours degree as well as my licence to practise. When I was first looking at acupuncture as a subject to study, I was not aware of the differences between styles and it was purely through luck and good fortune that I picked this form. I was immediately drawn to the Chinese Five Elements; I could instantly see how everything about them made such good sense, both from an acupuncture point of view and also in daily living.

From my early days in practice, I was always interested in facial and/or cosmetic acupuncture and the possibilities that it can offer for improvements to the skin's structure and facial suppleness. I started by experimenting with different facial points and looking at the results that could be achieved by their application. I was amazed at how, with continuous use of some points, the facial muscles could be trained, very similar to having a work-out in a gym. This change in the face remained for quite some time after treatment. The target was then to try to maintain these results long term.

With my Five Element Acupuncture training, I was fortunate to be able to incorporate body points into my treatments which helped to endorse and maintain the facial work that I was carrying out. I was also able to use my experience in this area to maximise the overall health and wellbeing of the patient, so that the effects were more far-reaching than appearance alone. As the treatments progressed, I began to use other needle techniques that would encourage the stimulation of collagen in the face and help to reduce fine lines and wrinkles. This combination of treatments resulted in a very powerful form of acupuncture, specifically developed for the face; this is what we call Facial Enhancement Acupuncture (FEA).

FEA continues to develop and is now practised in many countries throughout the world, with acupuncture practitioners attending our workshops and online courses on a weekly basis. However, it does not stop there; I am still making advancements in FEA and looking at new forms of needling for the face. These include techniques like Micro Needle Therapy (MNT), laser therapy and other forms of collagen induction.

I originally wrote *The Pocket Guide to Facial Enhancement Acupuncture* in 2006; this book was very well received, but covered only the basics of a FEA treatment. For some time, I have been looking forward to writing a far more comprehensive publication and I hope this is it; this book should cover all the basic information that an acupuncturist wanting to learn facial acupuncture needs to know.

This is by no means the end of the story; in fact, we are only just getting started. I am still amazed on a daily basis by the power of acupuncture, and facial acupuncture is no exception. FEA will continue to develop and I am excited about the prospects for its future.

CHAPTER 1

INTRODUCTION TO FACIAL ENHANCEMENT ACUPUNCTURE

As a Classical Five Element Acupuncturist, this form of treatment influences all that I do. You may already be familiar with the Chinese Five Elements of Wood, Fire, Earth, Metal and Water. Perhaps you are a practitioner of Five Element Acupuncture. However, there is no need to worry if you are not – knowledge of this style of acupuncture is not required to carry out a Facial Enhancement Acupuncture treatment. Having said that, I would like to give you a brief introduction to the Five Elements and show how they might be able to help you when treating a patient, be it for a conventional acupuncture session or a Facial Enhancement Acupuncture treatment.

1.1 THE FIVE ELEMENTS

The basis behind a Five Element Traditional Diagnosis is to try to work out which Element is your patient's Causative Factor (CF); this is the Element that remains with them from birth, or early childhood, for the rest of their life. The CF represents a person's underlying imbalance and once you have determined this Element, you can tailor your treatment plans with this in mind. In my experience, this additional information should help you to achieve some remarkable results.

Five Element practitioners diagnose a patient's Element by using four key factors: emotion, colour, odour and the sound of their voice. And, as we will see, the Five Elements of Wood, Fire, Earth, Metal and Water are also associated with, amongst other things, the organs of the body and the seasons. These correspondences extended to flavours, as outlined in this extract from the most significant book in the history of Chinese medicine, the *Nei Jing* (*Nei Ching*) or *The Yellow Emperor's Classic of Internal Medicine*:

> Hence if too much salt is used in food, the pulse hardens, tears make their appearance and the complexion changes. If too much bitter flavour is used in food, the skin becomes withered and the body hair falls out. If too much pungent flavour is used in food, the muscles become knotty and the finger and toe nails wither and decay. If too much sour flavour is used, the flesh hardens and wrinkles and the lips become slack. If too much sweet flavour is used in food, the bones ache and the hair on the head falls out. (Veith 1972, p.141)

Salt is the flavour of Water, bitter relates to Fire, pungent is associated with Metal, sour is linked to the Element of Wood and sweet correlates to Earth. This excerpt alone demonstrates how knowledge of the Five Elements can reveal a direct correlation to the condition of the skin and appearance.

Now, obviously I cannot explain in a few paragraphs what takes many years to learn, but I would like to give you a short taster of the Chinese Five Elements and how they may be incorporated into a Facial Enhancement Acupuncture treatment. You might then decide to explore the Five Elements further and in greater depth.

According to Taoist theory, the Five Elements were born of Yin and Yang and in turn they gave birth to the Ten Thousand Things. Many would say that this subject is a life-long study but, if this ancient classic is anything to go by, it is one well worth dipping in to for matters of longevity:

> This knowledge of the Tao and the workings of Yin and Yang was considered even strong enough to counteract the effect of age. Thus we find it said in the *Nei Ching* that 'Those who have the true wisdom remain strong, while those who have no wisdom grow old and feeble.' (Veith 1972, p.17)

To begin, let us look at each of the Five Elements individually.

1.1.1 THE WOOD ELEMENT

Spring is the season of the Wood Element, the time of rising Yang energy, creativity and birth:

> *Simple and fresh and fair from winter's close emerging,*
> *As if no artifice of fashion, business, politics, had ever been,*
> *Forth from its sunny nook of shelter'd grass – innocent, golden,*
> > *calm as the dawn,*
> *The spring's first dandelion shows its trustful face.*

> *(Whitman 1888, p.375)*

The spring is the time when we look forward to the coming year with optimism and excitement, or rather we should, if our Wood Element is in balance. This season is all about fresh starts and new things bursting into existence; it is seen in the plants and the trees around us and the wildlife coming to life after the long sleep of winter. We should be starting to make plans for the future now, putting to rest memories from the past and looking forward with optimism:

> Spring is the time of birth and regeneration. The burst of activity which surges out of the stillness of the winter has no equal elsewhere in the year; there is an energy and dynamic force abroad which brings life and vigour to everything. (Worsley 1998, p.1.2)

The spring can be a very lively and noisy time with people starting to go about their business and planning for the new year ahead. The animals are beginning to show more activity in the fields, as the spring lambs bounce around. It is generally a time when things start to happen after the shutdown of the winter months. The gift of this season is the optimism and chance to look to the future. It brings to us an opportunity to start again, to put failure behind us and take a fresh approach to life. Obviously, this only works if we are in balance. If we are suffering from an imbalance during this season, we will find it very hard to plan or look forward; we will have no energy, no drive and no ambition. If we have no vigour, then we can become depressed and anxious; these are all signs that something is not right.

Spring is linked with the Wood Element because of the prospects for growth and development. If a tree is not nourished and given a chance to grow, then it will wither and die, very much like the Body and also the Spirit of a person who is suffering from an imbalance. Again, like a tree, we must be able to bend and be flexible, adapting to things that may come our way. We must stay strong and rooted, but supple enough to give a little, should the need arise:

> And so the tree grows according to its destiny, in harmony with the seasons, in constant battle with the natural forces. As it grows strong, the winds and weather do it less harm. The tree maintains enough flexibility to sway in the wind, yet stays firmly rooted in the ground. (Herrmann 2000, p.180)

The Wood Element will show itself as someone who is well motivated and organised, someone who is a scrupulous planner; perhaps they might be self-employed or a director of a company, a person used to having life mapped out ahead of them. They are people who like to be pushed and their abilities tested and stretched. A Wood Element will be totally dedicated to anything that he or she pursues. This may be to do with work or the family; it can be taken literally to the point where that person would lay down their life for that cause. If we look at an historical example, we could see this devotion in Joan of Arc who, being so totally dedicated to what she believed in, became a martyr.

The spring is truly a time for inspiration, when everything looks more positive than perhaps at any other time of the year. This is the time when we can achieve and get things done:

> My beloved spake, and said unto me, Rise up, my love my fair one, and come away. For, lo, the winter is past, the rain is over and gone; The flowers appear on the earth; the time of the singing of birds is come, and the voice of the turtle is heard in our land; The fig tree putteth forth her green figs, and the vines with the tender grape give a good smell. Arise, my love, my fair one, and come away. (Song of Solomon 2:10–13, King James Version)

The emotion that is linked with the Wood Element is that of anger or lack of anger. When a Wood Element is in balance, this emotion will not necessarily be portrayed as the usual idea of anger, but perhaps more as a forcefulness of wanting to get things done, not tolerating laziness or sloppiness. Whereas a lack of anger will come across as someone who is very timid, and they may appear to have had the stuffing knocked out of them.

The sound that relates to this Element is that of shouting and patients with a constitutional imbalance may have a clipped or loud voice:

> The voice of thunder is heard and through the Spring Equinox, the *yang* makes its victorious rise more visible. Celebrations are in the making and everyone is excited, pushed on with a slight feverishness. The songs of the workers rise in harmony with this awakening of spring. These are the aspects of the second month: the Awakening of Insects and the Spring Equinox. (Larre 1994, p.28)

The Yin and Yang of this can be seen in the patient who may struggle to be heard.

1.1.2 THE OFFICIALS OF THE WOOD ELEMENT

Within each Element there are organs, also known as Officials, which process, store and distribute vital energy. Their functions are very specific and it is this, rather than the physical properties of each, that works to maintain life.

The Wood Element has two Officials: the Liver and Gall Bladder. They can be likened to the architect and the site foreman on a building site: one makes the plans and the others make the decisions on how to put these plans into progress.

Liver

The Liver is the 'Official of Planning'; this manifests itself in the Body, Mind and Spirit. We must all have a plan, be it long term or short term; otherwise we would lack direction and meander aimlessly. The Liver Official is always evident in a Wood Element as they are very serious planners. They usually have everything mapped out to the finest detail; they will also have a contingency plan prepared for those times when things do not go quite as they expected. A Wood Element in balance will have all the angles covered. When things are planned to this degree, it can give us the peace of mind to be able to relax, as we know we have all eventualities under control.

The Body has many contingency plans of its own that spring into action when they are required. When we cut ourselves, a plan is launched that begins to clot our blood. There are many plans that are in place, which release hormones into our system when our reserves are becoming depleted. Another example of a plan, this time solely in women, is that of the menstrual cycle. This is a plan that is regular when we are in balance; as soon as we suffer an imbalance these plans go out of the window and the menstrual cycle can become irregular or can even cease.

The Liver carries on planning for our futures and without this service we would flounder and lose direction. This Official also gives us the power to be flexible; when things do not quite go to plan, the Liver will give us the adaptability to change them. When there is an imbalance, any change of strategy, such as this, would be devastating and we would not be able to cope. The ability to plan is more important than ever to our Spirit; we need to be able to look to the long term and we want to be able to realise the goals that we have set for ourselves. Without this capacity to organise our lives and look ahead, it could almost feel as if we have no reason to exist.

The Liver is the Official responsible for managing the flow of Qi and also Blood. An imbalance would emanate in the Mind as an inability to move forward, a feeling of being stuck in the same place and eventually becoming stagnant, as nothing is moving. On a more physical level, an imbalance may show in the form of anaemia or some other blood disorders. It may also be evident in poor circulation, as the blood is not flowing freely to the extremities of the body. This in turn can cause poor joint conditions and arthritis. Also the nails on the fingers and toes usually show signs of being in a poor condition; these are obviously at the extremities and not receiving the circulation that is required.

Gall Bladder

> The gall bladder weighs 3 liang and 3 chu, is 3 ts'un long and lies within the shorter leaf of the liver... It can hold 3

ho of liquid essence (bile). The gall bladder's spirit is *Lung Yao* 'splendor of the dragon,' its epithet is 'the stately and the radiant one,' and its shape is that of a hybrid of turtle and snake. (Wallnofer and Von Rottauscher 1965, pp.82–84)

The Gall Bladder is the 'Official of Decision Making and Judgement'. It is the Official that converts the plans into actual decisions; it excels in making choices. Of course, if this Official is suffering from an imbalance, then the opposite applies and decisions will be very difficult to make.

Our whole existence involves decision making on one level or another. On the physical side, for every movement that we make, a decision has to be made as to which direction, or how much weight, or when can that arm or leg move. That is why people whose Gall Bladder is not functioning correctly might show signs of movement disabilities or stiffness of the joints. Obviously, decision making is more evident in a Mind situation, and without this Official functioning to its best capability, the person will stagnate and be unable to make any decisions – they will flounder without any direction or purpose. They may also resort to being very judgemental about others; they will have a fixed idea of how they think things should be and there is no room for reason or discussion over the matter.

The Gall Bladder is one of the most influential Officials in the body, becoming involved with all of the others; it directs and organises the rest: 'In Chinese medicine the Gall Bladder is said to be the only Official who works with pure essence; all of the others either store or come into contact with polluted or dirty energy' (Worsley 1998, p.10).

Western medicine sometimes removes the Gall Bladder in cases of disease and the patient can live a normal healthy life, but if that is the case, why do we have the organ in the first place? From this perspective, the Gall Bladder carries out the function of storing bile, which it regulates to the Small Intestine. Without the Gall Bladder the bile still flows to the Small Intestine, but in more of a drip-feed manner, rather than a regulated flow. Personally, I think I will try to retain my Gall Bladder. This decision follows what I, and medical doctors, considered to be a recent Gall Bladder issue. I had been experiencing some considerable pain under my ribs in the area of the Gall Bladder and after some treatment with acupuncture and adjustments to my diet I paid a visit to the doctor. They agreed with the diagnosis and I was sent for various scans and tests. The curious thing was that during the whole time I was suffering with the pain, my decision-making process had gone to pieces; a 'headless chicken' comes to mind – I could not make a decisive decision about anything.

Following the scans and regular acupuncture, my Gall Bladder had settled down and I felt quite strongly that, given the choice, I would not want to part with mine and face a life of indecisiveness.

1.1.3 THE WOOD ELEMENT FACIAL PATIENT

'The amazing ability of the liver to regenerate following partial resection or injury is unique, especially because the highly differentiated functions of the organ are totally maintained' (Papadimas *et al.* 2012, p.1). The qualities of regeneration held by the Liver are so important, especially from the perspective of ageing.

One thing that we can be sure of when we see a Wood patient for a Facial Enhancement Acupuncture treatment is that they would most likely have done their homework; they will know what they are looking for and will have everything planned to the finest detail. There should be no problems with this patient making a decision, unless of course they are out of balance and, if that is the case, perhaps some general acupuncture should be the first course of action.

One of the main symptoms in a Wood Element can be poor circulation, which means blood is not flowing freely to the extremities. This could manifest in the face and the skin; it may look dull and lifeless and there may be signs of age spots and discolouration. A Wood patient would definitely benefit from the circulatory stimulation that a Facial Enhancement Acupuncture treatment would bring to the skin.

1.1.4 THE FIRE ELEMENT

The Fire Element is linked to early summer, south and the colour red: 'Insects dart and buzz continually until the air itself seems to be in motion, while butterflies duck and rise like flames. Through it all, light and heat bear down with an intensity that sears the senses' (Reichstein 1998, p.52). This is the time of maximum Yang and the Fire Element CF will carry echoes of this in what is likely to be a passionate, friendly, enthusiastic and compassionate nature. The sun, at its zenith at this time of the year, fills us with warmth. The Fire Element has the power to transform things and this season has that quality: 'The term "fire"…also means "to transform"… the yang Qi are in charge and the ten thousand beings undergo change and transformation…' (Rochat de la Vallee 2009, p.71).

Often with a rosy or red complexion, the Fire person's dominant emotion is joy. Like the emotion of anger for Wood, this can manifest at either extreme as an excess of joy or a lack, leading to sadness. Problems in relationships can also derive from an out-of-balance Fire Element, either from not letting others in or by being too open, without determining whether someone is trustworthy.

A Fire CF is likely to be naturally tactile, flirtatious and at times inappropriate in what they say. When they are in balance, they can be happy, playful, great communicators and full of genuine laughter. It is then that this Element has the ability to truly listen to the needs of people in their lives.

1.1.5 THE OFFICIALS OF THE FIRE ELEMENT

Unlike the other Elements, the Fire Element has four Officials: Heart, Small Intestine, Pericardium and Triple Heater.

Heart

The Heart is the 'Supreme Controller' and that is exactly what it does; this Official should be protected at all costs. All of the other Officials are likened to the ministers in a court, who take their orders and allotted duties from the Heart. The Western medical view of the Heart is very important, but it is only really considered to be a pump. The Chinese perspective is far greater; you rely on your Heart to instruct the other Officials in the tasks that they should carry out, but these can only be the wishes and desires of the other Officials.

The Heart is also the home to our *Shen*. This is our Spirit. When our *Shen* is strong, this will show in our whole presence, the way we act and conduct our lives. Governing the distribution of Blood throughout the body, the Heart, when its flow is strong, will reach every corner of our physical being:

> Shen...is Yin in character and said to correspond to the mind. It is responsible for complex mental, emotional and spiritual feelings and affecting areas like consciousness, mental activities, memory, thinking and sleep. It receives its input from the senses, thus the events outside the body are directly related to a change in Heart rate. (Herrmann 2000, p.213)

The other view of the Heart is that of the Official of love and other emotions. This is very clear when traumas and feelings are evident. We are always hearing how the Heart was broken or how someone has given their Heart to someone. The Heart may be the Supreme Controller, but it is also very vulnerable to attack from the emotions and needs to be protected at all times.

Small Intestine

The Small Intestine is known as the 'Official Who Separates Pure from the Impure'. It is the Sorter.

The Stomach passes on the rotted and ripened food to the Small Intestine, whose role is to extract the pure Qi energy and then pass on the waste to the Large Intestine for disposal. This sorting helps to maintain a pure Mind and Spirit. If this Official is not functioning properly, it may become evident, in extreme cases, in depraved or degrading behaviour. The Small Intestine's link to Fire is that this Element helps to warm the positive Qi energy, to give warmth and joy to our lives.

There may be times when things seem confused and in a mess; this can be a sign that the Sorter is not working correctly. On a physical level, the Body can then become sluggish and slow; it becomes bogged down with bile and rubbish that is not being sorted by the Small Intestine. The stagnation of waste within the Body can show in the symptoms of a tummy ache, especially in children, or as pains, such as in the lower back. If this Official is not functioning properly, it can lead to stagnation or pollution not only of the Body but of the Mind and the Spirit too.

Pericardium

Also known as the 'Circulation Sex' and the 'Heart Protector', it protects the Supreme Controller from insult and injury. The Heart is so busy organising the other Officials that it does not have the time to watch its own back. That is where the Pericardium comes in; it is the bodyguard to the Heart.

The Heart Protector stands in the way when we suffer from physical or mental shocks:

> The Heart Protector's role should not come as a surprise to us since there are many parallels in nature around us of the same function. The bees protect their queen with millions of workers, so that she can be allowed to do her work without fear of invasion and attack. Herds gather themselves around their leader, and fend off threatening attacks. (Worsley 1998, p.11.3)

Triple Heater

The Triple Heater, also known as the Sanjiao or Triple Burner, is the 'Official in Charge of the Three Burning Spaces' within the main trunk of the Body. The interesting thing about the Triple Heater is that it is the only Official that does not manifest itself in any particular organ. It has a title, but no form as such; it is still an immensely important Official within the system. The main job of the Triple Heater is to maintain an even balance of heat across the three main areas of the Body; this sustains an even climate for each of the other Officials to perform at their optimum level. The nickname for this Official is the Heating Engineer; picture him running around your system maintaining the organs' output and reliability. If this Official becomes out of balance and too much heat accumulates, this can cause lethargy and laziness. Also, the Mind and Spirit start to overheat and we lose our tempers and patience. If it goes the other way and we begin to freeze, then things will eventually grind to a complete stop.

This Official also monitors the conditions that are around us; either in the climate or those that we may subject ourselves to, like hot baths or cold drinks, it then adjusts our Body's thermostats to suit.

So, although this Official has no form, its presence is felt throughout the Body; if it is sick and not performing its duties properly, then the whole system of Officials will cease to work correctly.

1.1.6 THE FIRE ELEMENT FACIAL PATIENT

'Facial complexion, which is a direct reflection of blood circulation, is also a major external indicator of heart function' (Reid 2001, p.55). Therefore, the Heart is indicated when the face shows excessive redness or, where there is a lack of Fire, an extremely pale complexion.

The Heart also houses the *Shen* and, as this links to the emotions, when troubled this can have an effect on stress levels and a patient's sleep. We all know how sleep deprivation (SD) can affect the way we look and feel, and a 2010 article collected data that shows why this may be happening:

> …reduction of sleep time seems in many ways to affect the composition and integrity of various systems. The SD causes an increased production of glucocorticoids, which may alter the integrity of the skin. In addition, the SD causes deregulation of the immune system, which consequently may also affect the integrity of collagen fibres. (Kahan *et al.* 2010, p.536)

We can see that the Fire Element out of balance can manifest in insomnia, which clearly can have a direct effect on the skin.

The emotion for Fire is joy and the sound is laughter. The focus of a Fire CF's treatment may even be around the fine lines and wrinkles that have formed from all that smiling. Like the sun, a Fire Element CF may like to be centre of attention. There is an underlying vulnerability that sees them hankering for compliments. This craving could be a driving force for them seeking treatment to enhance their appearance and is something that may come to light during the initial consultation.

1.1.7 THE EARTH ELEMENT

The Earth Element is linked to late summer, the time of declining Yang. Traditionally, it is seen as the central pivot for the other Elements: 'The exceeding beauty of the earth, in her splendour of life, yields a new thought with every petal' (Jefferies 2010, p.64).

An Earth Element is a person who is used to serving others. It is something they do without complaint and they are at their happiest when they are helping people with one thing or another. This rushing around looking after other people could lead to a feeling of emptiness, or being unfulfilled in one's self, because all of their energy and time is taken up by other people. This lack of fulfilment may manifest itself in an Earth Element as an eating disorder – a need to eat in order to give themself some attention. Although they would be eating, it would not necessarily be for the reasons of nutrition, but more than likely as a need to do something for themselves. This would probably lead to excessive eating and digestion problems, with a feeling of being bloated – an Earth Element may show signs of heaviness or lethargy.

Another sign of an imbalance in an Earth Element is for them to go to extremes of one form or another. They may become obsessed with cleanliness or with how they look, or they may go completely the opposite way and let their appearance and standards go altogether, not taking any interest in themselves at all. For some, these feelings go back to when they were children and their mother was always making sure that they were constantly clean, neat and tidy: 'The Earth Element nourishes us as our Mother, feeding and supporting us, giving us the ability to care for ourselves and others' (Worsley 1990, p.21). Of course, if this nurture was lacking in childhood, it can lead to a constant search for this kind of attention. When we understand this, it is not hard to see how the emotion associated with Earth is that of sympathy. This need can be excessive or there can be a complete lack of compassion.

We are all made up of the Five Elements and, although you may not consider your patient's primary CF to be Earth, you may recognise a little of this Element in their make-up. For example, they may feel that they are always taking on other people's problems or worrying about others and what might happen if they do not help them. There is often a fear of letting others down and, for an Earth Element, this can feel as if they are carrying a large weight across their shoulders, which stops them from walking upright and grinds them down. It is important for those with an Earth CF to realise that they can still care about people, but they need to take time to look after themselves too.

1.1.8 THE OFFICIALS OF THE EARTH ELEMENT

The Earth Element is all about nourishment and nurturing, about taking on board food and digesting and distributing it around the Body. This is done by the two Officials – the Stomach and the Spleen. As well as nourishing the Body we must also look after the Mind and Spirit equally.

Stomach

We must always be looking to digest as much knowledge as we can in order to keep the brain as active as possible. By absorbing this information, we are making ourselves feel secure and able to cope with problems. So, it is understandable that, when an Earth Element is out of balance, this can also affect the Mind. There will, of course, be the more obvious physical symptoms, but it will affect the Mind in similar ways to the Body. When the latter is not working correctly, the Stomach can feel knotted up and not able to receive any more nourishment. It is in this same way that the Mind and the Spirit can feel overwhelmed and unable to take any more in. It can become confused and discard information in a similar manner to the Stomach rejecting things when it is not right. These are all symptoms which demonstrate that both the physical and mental aspects of an Earth Element are not in balance.

The Stomach is referred to as the 'Official of Rotting and Ripening Food and Drink'; it digests the food that it receives and also controls the creation of waste by-products. We have observed that when something is out of balance it can affect the Mind as well as the Body. Someone with a Stomach imbalance may have a very vacant look about them, and they are unable to digest any facts or information that may be provided; this information will have to be condensed and fed to them in small sections so that they are able to take these facts on board. If too much information is thrown at them, they will show signs of confusion and also anxiety.

Spleen

The products processed by the Stomach, either nutritious or waste, are transported throughout the body by the 'Official of Transportation and Distribution' – the Spleen. If there is a breakdown or imbalance in these Officials, then the whole cycle of creation and distribution breaks down, thus creating problems throughout the whole Body and Mind. Both the

Stomach and Spleen are integral to the wellbeing of all of the other Officials throughout the body. In his book *In the Footsteps of the Yellow Emperor* (Eckman 1996, p.78), the author refers to ancient Chinese beliefs that the Stomach and Spleen Officials should be strengthened as a basis for all other treatments. If the distribution system is not functioning smoothly, then food and by-products will not be distributed and they will rot and cause blockages throughout the system; these Officials must be allowed to transport and distribute efficiently in order to maintain an even balance:

> Some readers may think that the image of a road haulage system does not do justice to the wisdom and beauty of this system of medicine, but in truth there is no better example from our daily lives than this. When food has been harvested, stored, or brought to market, it has to be taken to where it is needed as soon as possible or it will rot. Exactly the same applies within the body, mind and spirit. (Worsley 1998, p.13.7)

As with the Stomach, a similar distress can manifest itself when the Official of the Spleen is imbalanced. The Spleen is the transporter and, if this function is not working smoothly, worry and stress can set in, which can cause as much of a problem as a physical slow down or blockage in the Body.

From my studies of the Earth Element and its Officials, it has become clear that they are integral to the efficient running and maintenance of our Mind, Body and Spirit. The Stomach is the furnace that keeps our engines well stoked and full of power and energy – both for our physical wellbeing and to keep our Mind and Spirit alert. The Spleen provides the means for transporting this energy around our system to all the areas that require this stimulation. It seems evident that we would not be able to carry on with a healthy and rewarding existence if either of these Officials were not working correctly. Therefore, it must be in all of our interests to maintain a balance here before we can even look at other areas of our wellbeing.

1.1.9 THE EARTH ELEMENT FACIAL PATIENT

A deficiency in the Spleen will be indicated by sagging skin and a loss of tone to the face as this organ relates directly to the flesh: 'The Spleen controls the flesh' and 'flesh that is particularly flaccid or drawn, reflect imbalances in the spleen function' (Reichstein 1998, pp.105–106).

The Earth Element from a Facial Enhancement Acupuncture perspective is very interesting. Earth Elements can be obsessive about their appearance, so may be unrealistic about their expectations of what might be achieved by a facial treatment. This needs to be taken into consideration when you are discussing the expected results. When we look at the other side of an Earth imbalance, the patient may let themselves go and have no interest in how they look or what might be done to improve their skin or their appearance. The problem with this imbalance, of course, is that the patient is very unlikely to seek help through a Facial Enhancement Acupuncture procedure.

1.1.10 THE METAL ELEMENT

The Metal Element is linked to autumn, the time of rising Yin. Metal is about connection, inspirational quality and purity. Autumn is considered to be the time of winding down, getting together a storehouse ready to see you through the winter. If you do not get the reserves together in autumn, then it will be a very difficult winter to get through. It is also a time of reflection, when one looks back and perhaps takes stock of things and issues that have happened in the past. It can be a period when a person may paint or put their thoughts on paper and want to leave a more permanent record to pass on to their children and family. This can sound a little bit sombre, but it is not like that at all. Autumn is also the time when nature has a last burst of colour and energy, as the trees and plants give an exhibition of wonderful hues:

> Autumn in New England brandishes the changes of the season. Leaves turn vibrant colors, signifying the point of a cycle wherein all things begin to conserve and store themselves inside for nourishment, while externally life seems to be fading. (Connelly 1975, p.64)

The related emotion for this Element is grief. Those who experience a Metal imbalance may lose their judgement about when to let go and will often suffer from symptoms such as diarrhoea or constipation. The latter extreme can manifest in the Mind as an inability to let go and look forward; this person will always be thinking of what has gone before and perhaps what might have been. Like trees in autumn, they need to release their fruit and let it drop to the ground. What they are doing is hanging on and this fruit is rotting and causing them an imbalance.

It is very true that this time of the year is a period for reflection and we may all find ourselves looking back and contemplating whether the year has lived up to our expectations. It is very hard not to dwell on the past, but this is really wasted energy unless we can change our perspective of those events in order to move forward. What we need to do is look to the future and be positive in our attitudes, which is sometimes easier said than done.

Metal is attributed with discernment and quality and also purity; this can be likened to the rich minerals and ore that are found within the earth, which in turn can be processed to extract precious metals such as gold. These types of qualities in a person are something very special to have. They will come across, perhaps, as a perfectionist or as someone who wants things done properly and in order. They will likely be outspoken about their beliefs and have very high ethical and moral views:

> When minerals or ore are purified in intense heat, they give us the most precious substance, such as gold and diamonds. Yet often not only heat is needed for this process, but pressure, intense pressure that forces them to contract. The humorous remark that a diamond is just a piece of coal is perfectly accurate. They are both the same mineral i.e. carbon, yet one has been under heat and pressure and contracted infinitely more than the other. Similarly air in our lungs changes under pressure; some oxygen is removed, the air we breathe out is condensed. (Hermann 2000, p.107)

Air is also linked with the Element of Metal and obviously this is one of the greatest gifts that we have, as without it there would be nothing. Air is what gives us life and vitality and what feeds our lungs. We must be continually looking for that clean, fresh air that we require to develop and go forward.

We do not want to become bogged down with impure and stale air, which can be likened to the old memories and feelings from our past that may stop us progressing.

As we have discussed, a Metal Element is very pure and inspirational, someone who is organised and straightforward. As Earth relates to the mother, Metal is associated with the father, which speaks of authority and respect. This CF is likely to see things as cut and dried and would not want to see a 'do not care, do it tomorrow' type of attitude. You could sum it up by saying that you know where you stand with a Metal Element. Therefore, a challenge to someone of this Element would be disorganisation and irresponsibility; they would find it very difficult to tolerate scruffiness. Of course, as we have seen with each of the Elements, an imbalance could result in the other exaggeration, where someone could lose their self-esteem and become completely unkempt.

1.1.11 THE OFFICIALS OF THE METAL ELEMENT

When we focus on the Metal Element, we need to look at the two Officials of the Lung, known as the 'Official Who Receives the Pure Qi from the Heavens' and the Large Intestine, which is recognised as the 'Official of Drainage and Dregs'. These Officials are interrelated, as one brings goodness and vitality into the Body and the other expels the waste and by-products from the Body: 'The functions of the Officials of the Metal Element are in many ways the easiest to follow; they share a great many similarities with the physical functions of their equivalent organs in Western physiology' (Worsley 1998, p.14.1).

Lung

The Lung is of the greatest importance to us. It is the first sign of life when we are born and it is also the last sign when we pass away. It takes the energy from the outside of the body to the inside. It acquires what sustenance it needs from the air it has inhaled and then expels what it does not need when it exhales. The Lung Official then circulates this vital energy throughout the Body, Mind and Spirit. It breathes fresh air and life into our whole being and it also gets rid of the stale and tainted air that resides within us. However, we do seem to take even the act of breathing for granted. We have to eat, drink and breathe to survive, but we would soon panic if we could not find some food or water to consume. And yet we can go for days without this nourishment, but we can only survive for a matter of minutes without air.

Do we really take much notice of the air that we take into our lungs? As a society we are always polluting what we take in. We inhale cigarettes, either by choice or secondarily by the environment that we find ourselves in. We are forever breathing in pollution from cars and factories and yet we often do not seem to think twice about the consequences. If, however, we eat one too many cream cakes, then it is as if the world has come to an end! Diving was a regular hobby of mine and, despite not participating in a dive for a few years, I keenly remember the renewed sense of appreciation it gave me for the capacity of my lungs:

> As soon as he leaves the surface and descends, a diver is exposed to an increasing partial pressure of nitrogen. At the same time the effects of nitrogen narcosis begin. At shallow depths the effects are mild, but as he descends the effects increase, altering his awareness of events and his own behaviour. The danger in nitrogen narcosis lies mainly in the effect it has on the diver's awareness. Like a drunk who refuses to believe he has had too much to drink, a diver with nitrogen narcosis may not accept that there is anything the matter with him. (Anon. 1991, p.100)

The Lung Official is crucial to throwing away rubbish as it expels the carbon dioxide that builds up in our bodies. This pollutant is harmful and deadly and it is very important that it is removed from our systems.

Large Intestine

The other Official associated with the Metal Element is the Large Intestine. The Large Intestine is the 'Official of Drainage and Dregs'. It is responsible for getting rid of unwanted material that can cause blockages and problems when things are not running smoothly. Of course, this also applies to the Mind and Spirit; if things are allowed to build up and are not cleared out on a regular basis, then they will rot and become stale. This can lead to the Mind and Spirit becoming clogged up and not able to move forward.

This Official is the dustman for all of the other Officials. When it is working properly and on time, then the rubbish is cleared away and everything can flow efficiently. If we think back a few decades to the refuse collector's strikes in the UK, we can remember the devastation that was caused as the rubbish began to build up in the streets for many weeks. The danger of disease became very serious and eventually society would have ground to a halt. This is what happens to the Mind, Body and Spirit if this Official is not functioning correctly. Eventually everything will seize up and stop working. Even when it eventually starts performing as it should, there will be a backlog to clear up. Therefore, a complete balance may take some time to achieve.

1.1.12 THE METAL ELEMENT FACIAL PATIENT

I consider the Metal Element one of the easiest to recognise in a prospective Facial Enhancement Acupuncture patient. The skin is often referred to as the 'third lung' and most skin disorders are related to an imbalance in this Element. The *Nei Jing* states that 'The Lungs are connected with the skin' (Veith 1972, p.140).

Also, as the 'Official of Drainage and Dregs', if the Large Intestine is imbalanced, this could manifest as spots and acne or general poor skin quality. The skin is generally the first place to show any signs when there are toxins or impurities in the Body, so this patient would benefit from treating the Lung and Large Intestine points as well as the Facial Enhancement Acupuncture treatment.

Dry skin can also point to an imbalance here: 'Dry Evil is caused by insufficient moisture in the air and is particularly damaging to the lungs. It prevails in autumn and is associated with the Elemental energy of Metal' (Reid 2001, p.71).

Although, these symptoms may superficially indicate a primary imbalance, it is important to remember that not everyone who exhibits skin disorders of this kind will automatically be classed as a Metal Element CF. We are each made up of all of the Five Elements and they have a complex effect upon one another, so these issues may be an indication of an imbalance at another point in the cycle. This nuanced approach will require a much more in-depth study than we are able to explore here but, if this has not formed part of your acupuncture background, it is enough for now to be aware of these Elemental relationships.

Perfection is attributed to this Element and a prospective facial patient with an imbalanced Metal CF may well be on a quest to achieve this. It is all the more important to address this in the initial consultation and manage their expectations carefully.

1.1.13 THE WATER ELEMENT

The Water is linked to winter, the time of maximum Yin, but its power cannot be underestimated:

> *Under heaven nothing is more soft and yielding than water.*
> *Yet for attacking the solid and strong, nothing is better;*
> *It has no equal.*
> *The weak can overcome the strong;*
> *The supple can overcome the stiff.*
> *Under heaven everyone knows this,*
> *Yet no one puts it into practice.*
> *Therefore the sage says:*
> *He who takes upon himself the humiliation of the people*
> *   is fit to rule them.*
> *He who takes upon himself the country's disasters deserves*
> *   to be king of the universe.*
> *The truth often sounds paradoxical.*
>
> *(Tsu 1972, ch.78)*

The type of character that first springs to mind when thinking about a Water Element is one of the guys in the classic movie *Easy Rider*. A rebel image conjures up the type of person that does not want to stay in one place for too long and is always looking to move on – someone who does not conform and stands out from the crowd.

If you can call it a gift, then it would be that a Water Element is a free spirit; any obstacle that confronts them is easily worked around, like a river finding its way around obstructions or boulders in its way. When balanced, they adapt to the shape that contains them, which, on the flip side, can indicate a need for boundaries, lest the Water overflows and loses control, using up their reserves.

In fact, the persona of a Water Element sounds like a very cool and attractive one to have, a bit of a James Dean figure, a person that is hard to pin down, who is perhaps on a different wavelength to the majority of people, but who risks depleting their Essence:

> Water itself is naturally elusive and resists definition. It can hold any shape, and yet cannot itself be grasped and held once and for all. It appears to have boundaries, and yet will find a passage around any dam or obstruction wherever it can. (Worsley 1998, p.6.1)

The emotion associated with the Water Element is that of fear, or lack of fear. This feeling can be traced back many years to when farmers would have built up their stores of grain and crops to last over the barren winter months. There was the fear that if this was not done, then there would be no food left come the spring. This fear is still evident today in Water Elements who, during the winter, are very conscious to conserve things and are frightened of the consequences if they do not. A farmer would be very careful to make sure that he conserved as much water as possible, so that there would be enough supply for the dry season to follow.

Take time to observe the relentless persistence of Water to get to where it wants. This is a feature that you can see if someone's Water Element is balanced; they will be persistent in what they do and not give up: 'Over time it can wear away the hardest rock and make it smooth' (Hicks and Hicks 1999, p.180).

Notice the smell. Each Element has an odour and Water's is putrid. The sound that is linked to the Water Element is that of groaning. This is very evident when you are taking a walk along the beach: the sea has that relentless groaning sound, one minute quiet and then a groan as the wave reaches a peak and breaks – a similar sound to a train. Finally, the taste associated with Water is salty, and of course you can taste this on your tongue very easily when you are near to the sea.

1.1.14 THE OFFICIALS OF THE WATER ELEMENT

These two Officials really do exactly what it says on the tin! They deal directly with the Water Element. Between them they govern the major aspects of our vital fluids. They are of the greatest importance to the whole of the Body and other Officials, as none of them can function without Water.

Kidney

The Kidney Official is known as the 'Official Who Controls the Waterways'. This, however, may be a little misleading as the Kidney does far more. Ancient Chinese philosophy believed that the Kidney Official was the storehouse for ancestral energy that was passed on to each generation; it was the seed of life that was handed down.

The Official takes some of the Qi energy from our consumption of food and air and compiles it as a reserve. This supply can be called upon when we have heavy physical or mental tasks to cope with. A part of the Kidney Official is the Ming Men. This is responsible for warming the Essence of the Kidney, and it is also a very important part of the Official as it is a warmer for all of the Body's organs.

The Essence that we have mentioned is called the Kidney *Jing*. This is derived from both pre- and post-Heaven Essence. The pre-Heaven Essence is inherited from our parents at conception. It can be gradually depleted throughout our lifetimes unless it is conserved well. The post-Heaven Essence is taken from food and nourishment and can be replenished.

The function of Kidney *Jing* in our bodies is to do with the basis of growth and development; deficiency can result in stunted growth or retardation and bone and teeth problems.

Kidney *Jing* is also the basis of our constitutional strength and the production of bone marrow, which fills the brain and the spinal cord. The pathology of someone with deficient Kidney *Jing* will be that of someone who is always weak and prone to constant infections.

Bladder

The Bladder is the 'Official Who Controls the Storage of Water' and it is the reservoir of the Body, Mind and Spirit. This is the reserve that we draw from in the winter when things are running low. If this is lacking, then things can start to go wrong in all three aspects.

As well as being a reservoir, the Bladder is also charged with disposing of the impurities found in our urine; if these are left to build up and not disposed of, this can eventually pollute our whole being.

So, if the Bladder is out of balance, it may not be able to keep its fluids within its boundaries. This may manifest as incontinence and cystitis-type infections. The Bladder is one of the few Officials that is similar in its description of use in both Chinese and Western medicine. It is also the longest meridian on the body with 67 points. The Bladder and the Kidney need to be looked at in the context of equal importance: 'The Kidneys are rulers over the winter. Kidneys and Bladder are related and have to be treated as one in acupuncture' (Wallnofer and Von Rottauscher 1965, p.90).

These two Officials of the Water Element need to be dealt with the greatest of respect, as they are responsible for a huge amount of water in the body – in fact, according to Masaru Emoto in his book *The Hidden Messages in Water*, 'the average human body is 70 percent water' (2004). That is a large volume of fluid that needs retaining and managing, so these organs need to be in the best of condition.

1.1.15 THE WATER ELEMENT FACIAL PATIENT

From a an emotional point of view, a Water Element patient looking at a Facial Enhancement Acupuncture treatment might express irrational fears, perhaps about growing old or the ageing process in general. They may be frightened by the prospect of so many needles and potential risks, so they will need more reassurance than most. Alternatively, they will exhibit a complete lack of fear and will seem unfazed. They may have even chosen to have this type of treatment because it is unconventional and appears daring. Whether terrified or unperturbed, you can be sure that, once they have begun, they will be determined to see the course of treatment through.

As we have seen, the Kidneys house our inherited energy or Essence. When this is strong, we will 'grow old gracefully', and if it is weak, 'old age may arrive prematurely' (Hicks and Hicks 1999, p.181) It is clear to see that strengthening and maintaining the Kidney *Jing* can help retain vitality and youthfulness.

The Bladder is also an important meridian in facial acupuncture, as the channel passes over both the head and face. This Official helps to expel impurities from the Body, so, again, similar to the Metal Element, there may be skin conditions such as greasy skin or blackheads that become evident when this Element is out of balance.

1.2 THE HISTORY OF FACIAL ACUPUNCTURE

At the beginning of the twentieth century, 1024 prescriptions left by medicine men were unearthed from the Mogoa Grottoes at Dunhuang situated along the Silk Road in China: 'Most of the manuscripts are from the Sui or Tang dynasties and give a variety of prescriptions', including literature about dermatology, and the 'experts were also attracted by a considerable number of cosmetic recipes such as facial creams, hair tonics and shampoos' (Feng and Zheng 1994, p.96).

These findings show evidence of China's long-held beauty tradition, but the practice of skin rejuvenation stretches back well before the arrival of the Sui (AD 589–618) and Tang (AD 618–907) Dynasties. For instance, the *Shan Hai Jing* or *Classic of Mountains and Seas* was written during the Warring States period (475–221 BC) and finalised during the Western Han Dynasty (206 BC–AD 9). It detailed many herbal preparations for skin problems and anti-ageing. Birrell's translation identifies some of these solutions, such as the fat from a goat-antelope that could be used to cure chapped skin and 'a bird on this mountain named the wagtail… It is effective for wrinkles' (Birrell 1999, p.13).

Believed to be authored in the Eastern Han Dynasty (AD 25–220) the *Shen Nong Ben Cao Jing* or 'The Divine Farmer's Materia Medica' was another well-known compilation detailing Chinese herbal medicines. Many of the preparations are recommended to slow ageing and prolong life and there are those, such as 'Bai Zhi', that offer skin rejuvenating properties: 'It promotes the muscles and skin and moistens and makes [the skin] shiny. It can be used to make a face cream' (Yang 1998, p.58)

The desire for skin enhancing seems clear and there is evidence that the acupuncture points of the face have been used for many years in Chinese medicine. The *Zhen Jiu Jia Yi Jing* or 'The Systematic Classic of Acupuncture and Moxibustion' was completed a few years before the arrival of the

Western Jin Dynasty (AD 265–317) by Huang-fu Mi (AD 214–282). This is one of the most influential books ever written on acupuncture as not only did it gather together information from the ancient *Ling Shu*, *Su Wen* and *Ming Tang*, but it also detailed acupuncture points, the channels and the clinical applications of treatment. Nine types of needle were introduced, including one specifically for treating the skin: 'The skin is associated with the lung and hence with a person's yang. Therefore, in treating of (the skin) the arrowhead needle (chan) is employed' (Yang and Chace 1994, p.162). The text discusses facial complexion and the condition of the hair as an indication of potential disease, due to particular imbalances in the body.

It is widely held that the Chinese empress, and the emperor's concubines, as far back as the Song Dynasty (AD 960–1279) received acupuncture to aid rejuvenation and specifically promote anti-ageing: 'A remarkable blossoming of acupuncture occurred under this dynasty. We owe this period the famous Bronze Man, the founding of a faculty of acupuncture and the printing and distribution of drawings and important works' (Soulie de Morant 1994, p.12). It was certain that huge advances were made during this dynasty and 'the Song emperors took a personal interest in acupuncture studies' (Soulie de Morant 1994, p.840). Wang Weiyi wrote some of the most notable books of the time and was charged by Emperor Ren Zong, who reigned from AD 1023–1064, with the task of studying 'the method of needles and moxa and to have a statue cast as a model' (Soulie de Morant 1994, p.840). Drawings were also made to pin down what was known about the points. The Emperor wanted the practice of acupuncture to be standardised and Wang Weiyi's Bronze Man was a valuable teaching aid. The model detailed the points of the face and could be used as a means to educate students about disorders of the skin and balancing the body to prolong life and the signs of ageing:

> Before the exam the model was covered with a thick layer of wax, which was then allowed to set so that the holes at the position of the acupuncture points could not be seen. The hollow interior of the model was then filled with water. A student would be told about a case and asked how he would treat it using acupuncture. After describing which points he would use and why, he was asked to locate them on the

> model and told to insert them, through the wax and into
> the hollows below so that, when the needles were removed,
> water would flow out. (Kidson 2008, pp.17–18)

The Emperor's endorsement would have seen the practice flourish and he, and his entourage, would no doubt have had a vested interest in the advancements of acupuncture available at the time.

The Ming Dynasty (AD 1368–1644) saw further development in cosmetology when Li Shi Zhen, one of the most highly regarded Chinese physicians in history, wrote the classic *Cao Gang Mu* or 'Materia Medica': 'Linking chapters to specific facial features, Li Shi Zhen addressed the unique treatment requirements of the eyes, nose, lips, teeth and hair, as well as the more overriding issues of complexion and wrinkles' (Zhang 2006, p.7). Related beauty techniques using jade rollers are also deemed to have their origins in this era. China's Forbidden City, built during the Ming Dynasty, is said to display them as part of the Emperor's bedroom necessities in the Imperial Palace.

Following this lengthy tradition, with its surge in popularity in the 1970s, acupuncture started to take its place in the West and interest grew as to the various benefits that could be obtained from treatment. (Meng, Xu and Lao 2011). In my experience, acupuncture points, both on the body and also the face, have always shown very good results in treating many conditions of the skin and also the facial muscles, particularly in the case of stroke patients and those demonstrating other muscular problems.

Acupuncture has been used to promote longevity, enhance the skin and reverse the signs of ageing for centuries. However, it is probably only in the past few decades that acupuncture points of the face have been used in any sequence with the goal of providing a full facial acupuncture treatment. The cosmetic acupuncture protocols, as we recognise them today, are now practised around the world. I am sure that they will continue to evolve and develop, but their roots will remain in the foundations of acupuncture established many hundreds of years ago.

1.3 MODERN-DAY TREATMENT COMPARISON

The results that are most expected from a facial acupuncture treatment are a smoothing of the skin and reduction in fine lines and wrinkles. From a Western point of view, at the time of writing, the nearest comparison would be with a Botox® treatment.

Botox® is one of the commonly used trade names for the neurotoxic protein called Botulinum toxin type A that is produced by the bacterium *Clostridium botulinum* (Benedetto 1999). As its name suggests, 'Botulinum toxin is one of the most poisonous substances known' (Barbano 2006, p.E17). However, once the same toxin is isolated and purified, it can be used for cosmetic purposes. The protein can then be used to treat such things as brow furrows, wrinkles and areas of the face like the nasal labial fold. The procedure involves a small amount of the diluted toxin that is injected into the area in question; this has the effect of freezing the muscles in order to prevent the wrinkle or crease forming. The Botox® protein acts by blocking the nerve impulses that contract the facial muscles; if the muscles can no longer contract, then the wrinkles will soften and become less pronounced. The effects of Botox® are not permanent and will generally only last for up to six months, after which time repeated treatments would then be required to prolong them.

As we mentioned earlier, we must remember that Botox® or Botulinum toxin is a poison. One way to get botulism is to eat something containing the neurotoxin produced by the bacterium *Clostridium botulinum*. A very serious symptom is paralysis, which in some cases can go on to become fatal. Obviously, the amounts that are used in a cosmetic procedure are diluted; there would be very little chance of any such effects, when administered by a professional. Still, we need to remember that Botox® is a toxin and it carries a number of potential side-effects.

Botox® and similar types of facial treatments are always going to prove popular with the public. They offer a quick fix and will give an instant outcome, and unfortunately contemporary society is one in which people expect results straight away. Facial acupuncture is a far more subtle, yet natural, approach to working with the face and, if your patients can be persuaded to wait a little longer for the results, I am sure they will be impressed. I have also found that as people's awareness grows and they begin to consider carefully what they are putting into their bodies, they become more switched on to a more natural approach to anti-ageing. Facial Enhancement Acupuncture offers this safe, holistic alternative.

1.4 THE DEVELOPMENT OF FACIAL ENHANCEMENT ACUPUNCTURE

So, although facial acupuncture can obtain similar effects to modern-day treatments, it is not a new idea. Despite having very little written about it in English, we can see that it is likely to have been in use for at least a millennium. With this ancient heritage in mind, I feel that we need to think of facial acupuncture, or cosmetic acupuncture as it is also known, as simply another form of acupuncture, an extension of what an acupuncturist already does.

As a Five Element Acupuncturist, I look after my patients by treating their Mind, Body and Spirit. By focusing on their face, I see this as an add-on to my existing acupuncture services.

I began to develop Facial Enhancement Acupuncture after considering the locations of the acupuncture points on the face and their positions, with reference to the facial muscles. I remember looking at one of my anatomy books, when I was studying, and thinking: 'Stomach 9 (ST9) is a fantastic point used in Five Element Acupuncture as a "Window of the Sky" point.' Combined with its location, with reference to the muscles of the neck, I began to question how needling this point might affect them. There are, of course, so many other acupuncture points with prominent positions on the face and yet the majority I would generally not use in my day-to-day acupuncture practice; points such as Stomach 3 (ST3) and Stomach 4 (ST4). Then we have the wonderful points around the eyes such as Bladder 2 (BL2) and Triple Heater 23 (TH23); these are great points that help with so many eye conditions. So, combining all of these points into a protocol means that we get to use these fantastic points each time we carry out a treatment.

Facial Enhancement Acupuncture quickly became an integral part of my own practice. I started to monitor the results that I was achieving using facial points and also developed different needle techniques to achieve results in other areas, such as targeting fine lines and wrinkles. It soon became clear that regular use of these facial points would have a profound effect on the facial muscles and achieve results that far outweighed my original expectations. My Facial Enhancement Acupuncture treatments now include various body points and auricular points that I have included in my protocol over the years. These additional points, although not situated on the face, can have a profound effect on your patient's appearance. The treatment plan is always evolving and I am continually looking at new points or techniques that will improve the overall Facial Enhancement Acupuncture treatment experience.

Facial Enhancement Acupuncture has grown rapidly and to date I have trained acupuncturists in over 30 countries worldwide and this is still growing year on year. It is a very simple concept and, aside from its holistic benefits, works on two main areas: the muscles of the face and the lines and wrinkles of the skin.

1.4.1 THE MUSCLES OF THE FACE

To begin, we will look at the muscles of the face. We can divide this into five simple muscle groups. With each of these sections, the technique is the same; we are stimulating these muscles by using our acupuncture needles. Think of the facial muscles going to the gym; we are giving each muscle a work-out by stimulating it with our needle.

These muscle groups are easy to remember: Eyes, Nose, Mouth, Jaw, and Neck. If we take a look at these five groups, we can see the muscles in relation to the face and visualise our point locations accordingly.

Eye Muscles

- *Corrugator supercilli*: Pulls the eyebrows together in a frown and is often paralysed with botulinum toxin (Botox®) to prevent development of wrinkles.

- *Frontalis*: Raises the eyebrows.

- *Orbicularis oculi*: Narrows the eyes to a squint.

- *Procerus*: Pulls the eyebrows down and together.

See Figure 1.1.

Nose Muscles

- *Depressor septi*: Depresses the nostrils.

- *Levator labii superioris alaeque nasi*: Flares the nostrils.

See Figure 1.1.

Mouth Muscles

- *Buccinator*: Helps form the cheeks to blow a kiss.

- *Depressor anguli oris*: Makes the lips grimace.

- *Depressor labii inferioris*: Makes the lips pout.

- *Levator labii superioris*: Opens the lips.

- *Mentalis*: Wrinkles the chin.

- *Orbicularis oris*: Helps the lips form a shape to whistle.

- *Platysma*: Pulls the corners of the mouth together.

- *Risorius*: Helps the mouth form a grin.

- *Zygomaticus major and zygomaticus minor*: Lift the mouth to smile.

See Figure 1.1.

Jaw Muscles

- *Masseter*: Clenches the teeth together.

- *Temporalis*: Raises the lower jaw when chewing.

See Figure 1.1.

Neck Muscles

- *Sternocleidomastoid*: A pair of muscles running down either side of the neck, which help to lift and rotate the head.

See Figure 1.1.

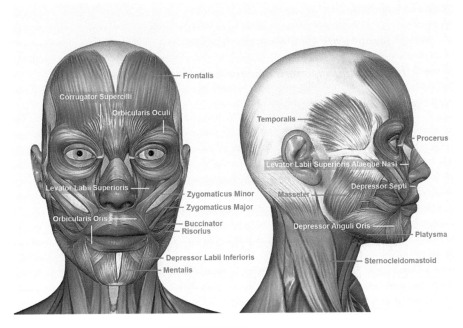

FIGURE 1.1 THE FACE AND NECK MUSCLES

We will cover the points used in a Facial Enhancement Acupuncture treatment in Chapter 3. For now, it is important to recognise that, by stimulating the acupuncture points on and near to these muscles, we will be affecting the overall appearance and tightness of the face.

1.4.2 LINES AND WRINKLES

The second main part of a Facial Enhancement Acupuncture treatment addresses the problems of fine lines and wrinkles. These become evident in most areas of the face as we get older, but can also be caused by excess sun and environmental conditions.

The technique we use for dealing with these areas is to use acupuncture needles directly into the line or wrinkle; this action creates a very small wound to the face which the body then endeavours to repair. As it does this, the body produces natural collagen and wound-healing properties which fill out the line, and with continued treatment the line or wrinkle should gradually fade. This same technique can also be successfully employed on age spots and old acne scars; in fact, any area of the face that requires collagen induction will benefit from the insertion of acupuncture needles into the area.

When I first developed Facial Enhancement Acupuncture, I used small intradermal needles to work on lines and wrinkles and we will cover the use of these needles later in the book. As technology develops and my experience of needling the face has grown, I am now looking at additional methods of addressing these areas. These make use of tools such as lasers and dermal rollers within the practice of Micro Needle Therapy. We will take a closer look at the latter new system as we progress, but we must always be aware that Facial Enhancement Acupuncture as a treatment protocol will continually develop as our expertise in this field grows.

I am sure that as your practice and use of Facial Enhancement Acupuncture advances, both you and your patients will be amazed at the results that can be achieved. Remember, however, that this is not a treatment that garners immediate results; a course of treatment is necessary, with regular maintenance. This will give your patients long-term sustainable results, which have been achieved totally naturally. What could be better than that?

CHAPTER 2

EXPECTED RESULTS OF FACIAL ENHANCEMENT ACUPUNCTURE

As soon as I mention Facial Enhancement Acupuncture to someone, either a friend or a prospective patient, you see their eyes light up and the majority reach for the neck and jowl area, expressing their excitement at the prospect of a facelift. That is all well and good and it is great that people are so enthusiastic, but we do need to make it clear to prospective patients that facial acupuncture is not a facelift, at least not in the context of what they might consider one to be. To understand a patient's expectations of a traditional facelift, we need to examine what exactly a facelift does.

A facelift, technically known as a rhytidectomy (literally meaning the surgical removal of wrinkles), will usually involve the abstraction of excess skin from the face and a tightening of the underlying tissues. This kind of invasive procedure to the patient's face and neck will carry the risks that any surgery would have.

With Facial Enhancement Acupuncture, we are working more to stimulate the muscles of the face and also to aid the production of natural collagen in the dermis. Targeting the muscles in particular will have an overall lifting effect but, with all the best intentions in the world and the most skilled acupuncturist, it is very unlikely that you will be able to achieve the results that would be attained by a surgical facelift. Therefore, it is very important to stress to your patient exactly what the treatment is you are offering and the expectation of results that can be achieved.

The secret of a successful and beneficial Facial Enhancement Acupuncture treatment is to manage the patient's expectations. When you first meet your patient, you will carry out a full consultation and it will soon become clear to you what they are looking for. From this first visit, you may find that their expectations are probably very unrealistic for the type of treatment that you are offering.

No matter how competent an acupuncturist you are or how experienced with carrying out facial acupuncture treatments, the reality is that most goals that patients are looking to achieve with a treatment will be beyond the reach of Facial Enhancement Acupuncture. I have found that the vast exposure to celebrities in the media can often result in very high expectations from patients. The trend for digitally enhancing images in magazines can also give unrealistic aims.

Having said all of that, I am not suggesting that Facial Enhancement Acupuncture will not provide your patients with some impressive results, because it most definitely will. It is important to remember to manage your patient's expectations; if you do this successfully, they will not be disappointed and you will have a happy patient who will return for further treatments.

When you first talk to your patient, ask them to describe to you what they think about their appearance. What would they like to change if they possibly could? Ask them to show you the area of the face that they are not happy with and make a note of their comments. You can look back after a few treatments and assess the progress that has been made. One thing that will quickly become apparent is that people will soon forget what they originally talked about, so it is always useful to be able to check back in the file and see what areas of the face you were targeting with your treatment.

When I have conducted consultations in the past, on a number of occasions it has become clear that the patient's expectations from the treatment are going to be more than we can accomplish with facial acupuncture. Using your skills as a therapist, you might determine from your consultation that the patient has deeper issues going on, perhaps emotionally rather than physically. These deep-rooted problems may have prompted them to look into changing their appearance. I would recommend discussing this further with your patient and deciding the appropriate line of treatment to take. It is well worth bearing in mind that, whatever results you might achieve for that patient, they are unlikely to be happy if there are underlying issues surrounding their need to alter the way they look.

Let us assume that you have carried out your consultation with your patient and they have outlined a few areas of the face that they would like to improve upon. What realistic results can be achieved by using Facial Enhancement Acupuncture? One of the most dramatic improvements that patients often report back to me is that the quality of their skin is vastly improved, even after only the first treatment. This is not surprising as we are directing a lot of Qi energy to the face. When you add the stimulation effect of the needles, this is improving circulation and blood flow to the skin's surface. This can, in turn, reduce redness and improve the overall definition of the skin. Another noticeable improvement is the reduction in puffiness of some areas of the face.

The two main areas of the face that are mentioned the most in a consultation are the lines between the eyes at the bridge of the nose and also the line that runs from the corner of the mouth to the edge of the nose – the 'nasal labial fold'. If, as a practitioner, we can do something about these, then we will have many happy patients. Facial Enhancement Acupuncture is very successful at reducing the appearance of lines in these two areas and you will find that, on most patients, they will achieve a very dramatic reduction in the line depth and severity after a few treatments.

Another area of the face that I am asked if I can improve is the eyes, especially drooping eyebrows, which tend to drag a person's face down. Facial Enhancement Acupuncture can be really effective in helping to lift a patient's eyebrows and we will cover the specific points that help to do this in Chapter 3.

So far we have been able to offer the patient improved skin quality and texture and also been able to reduce the depth and severity of lines on the forehead and to the side of the mouth; we have also been able to address the problem of drooping eyebrows.

The other area of concern to patients is often the jowls that we previously mentioned. This is probably one of the hardest areas of the face to treat, as so much can depend on other factors such as the patient's weight or general facial structure. If we look at the fat components of the cheek, we will see that there are two distinct overlapping fat compartments that are above and below the mandible bone. The *mandibular septum* separates the jowl fat in the cheek from the fat in the neck (Reece, Pessa and Rohrich 2008). What we can do with Facial Enhancement Acupuncture is start to try to tighten the muscles in the face and the neck in order to reduce the appearance of the jowls. It is surprising how effective this can be and, although it will never achieve the results of a surgical facelift, it might be all that is needed to improve this area of your patient's face.

In my clinic we have patients who come for a one-off treatment, perhaps in the build-up to a special occasion, and others who make Facial Enhancement Acupuncture a regular part of their beauty regime. With the latter, you should notice a very dramatic improvement in the appearance of any lines on the face and also the general tightness of the skin. With regular follow-up maintenance sessions, there should be no reason why this improvement cannot be sustained in the long term.

Of course, we must not forget that there are lots of other facial issues that we can address using traditional acupuncture. Your patient may express concerns about dark circles under their eyes or perhaps swelling around them and eye bags. These are all constitutional issues that we can tackle using acupuncture points of the face and the body. We will look at some of these conditions and treatments in Chapter 6 and you can consider their additional use in your treatments.

A one-off session is an ideal way to experience a Facial Enhancement Acupuncture treatment, but to obtain the best long-term results I would advise a course of ten treatments at weekly intervals. This can then be followed by regular one-month to six-weekly maintenance treatments. This treatment plan will give your patients the optimum results and endurance to the improvements that you have made.

To recap, it is of the upmost importance that you should manage your patient's expectations of their treatment. If you can do this successfully, you will have a satisfied patient.

CHAPTER 3

ACUPUNCTURE
POINTS USED IN THE
MAIN PROTOCOL

3.1 THE AGGRESSIVE ENERGY
TREATMENT (AE DRAIN)

The AE Drain, as taught by J.R. Worsley, is a treatment protocol that is used in Five Element Acupuncture to clear an accumulation of unhealthy Qi energy from a patient's system. This build-up of Aggressive Energy (AE) can have an external or internal cause and the Yin organs usually trap the heat from this resulting stagnation. In many of the ancient texts, it is thought that a build-up of Aggressive Energy can be extremely debilitating or even life-threatening.

The lineage of Five Element is thought to be an oral tradition dating back to the practitioner Liu Wan-Su (AD 1110–1200) and preserved in Taiwan. As Peter Eckman describes in *The Footsteps of the Yellow Emperor*, the concept of AE was brought to Europe by French acupuncturist Jacques Lavier from Taiwan, where he studied with Wu Wei-p'ing in the 1950s: 'whose treatment protocol calls for draining the AEP's (Back Shu Points) of the Zang Organs involved, prior to energetic balancing' (Eckman 1996, pp.147–150). This point is further elaborated:

> Li Dong-yuan, during the same epoch as Liu Wan-su, recommended a similar protocol – treating the Back Shu Points of the Zang Organs for any condition resulting from the penetration of environmental Evil Qi secondary to a deficiency of central Qi. (Yang and Li 1993 in Eckman 1996, p.150)

I like to use this protocol each time I see a new patient in the clinic and before we embark on a course of treatment. One AE Drain is usually sufficient to begin with, but sometimes we may have to go back and repeat the procedure later in the patient's course of treatment if problems do not appear to be clearing.

The following Back Shu points are used for clearing Aggressive Energy:

- BL13 Lung Shu

- BL14 Pericardium Shu

- BL15 Heart Shu

- BL18 Liver Shu

- BL20 Spleen Shu

- BL23 Kidney Shu.

Also, we need to use a couple of test needles that are inserted level with, or just outside of, the Bladder meridian. If Aggressive Energy is present, you will see redness around the base of the needles; this redness is also called erythema. The colour that emerges around the Back Shu points should be a darker red than at the test needles. This will confirm that your needle positions for the Back Shu points are correct. See Section 4.1 for the full AE Drain protocol.

3.2 ACUPUNCTURE POINTS ON THE FEET AND LEGS
LIVER 3 TAI CHONG (SUPREME RUSHING)

Location: Between the first and second metatarsals on the dorsum of the foot.

Element: Wood.

Functions: Spreads Liver Qi and Blood, also relieves pain. Subdues Liver Yang and calms anger.

Applications: Headaches, hypertension, eye problems, genital and gynaecological problems.

Liver 3 (LV3) is known as a Source point and each of the acupuncture meridians has its own. I have heard Source points likened to a main station on a train line. They are high-concentration points that provide access to the main meridian system.

LV3 has many uses in Chinese medicine, as outlined, and is a powerful point. It is a particularly useful point for feelings of being stuck. When needling LV3, there is usually a very strong sensation which can be felt in the foot and sometimes through the length of the leg along the Liver meridian.

STOMACH 36 ZU SAN LI (LEG THREE MILES)

Location: 3 cun below Stomach 35 (ST35), one finger width lateral from the anterior border of the tibia. (See Glossary for a definition of cun measurement.)

Element: Earth.

Functions: Restores balance to Qi, harmonises the Stomach, strengthens the Body and Spleen and enhances immune function.

Applications: Indigestion, stomach pain and vomiting.

Stomach 36 (ST36) is a very important point; enriching for Mind, Body and Spirit. Having this point needled often produces a strong sensation that sometimes travels down the leg. Most acupuncturists consider ST36 as a point that they would use for digestive issues; it is indeed a universal point that I would use for any condition from diarrhoea to heartburn. I would also consider using ST36 when the system needs a boost. Of course, if your patient lacks energy, this will often manifest in the face. The Stomach channel begins on the face and, according to a 2012 study, 'suspended moxibustion over Zusanli (ST 36) has a very significant increase in temperature at the forehead, around the nose, at the corners of the mouth, and at the cheeks and lips' (Yang *et al.* 2012, pp.397–403).

The Stomach channel descends from the face to the feet and ST36 is commonly used as an anaesthetic point, as we will discover in the next section. And, according to the theory of Tsang Fu Chinglo, 'Where the meridian passes, there is healing' (in Anon. 1974, p.77).

ST36 is also a He-Sea point, one of the connecting points found at the elbows and knees. Not only that, it is a strong Earth Element point responsible for nourishment and feeding the other organs of the body. Therefore, it is considered to be a significant point for general patient wellbeing.

SPLEEN 9 YIN LING QUAN (YIN MOUND SPRING)

Location: In the depression, distal and dorsal to the medial condyle of the tibia.

Element: Earth.

Functions: Expels dampness, strengthens the Spleen, restores balance to bodily fluids.

Applications: Menstrual problems, urinary retention, knee pain, chronic yeast infections and candida.

Spleen 9 (SP9) is a Water He-Sea point on an Earth channel. It is a very important point on the meridian for transportation and nourishment around the body, often used in conjunction with ST36. The Spleen is responsible for sending fluid up to the lungs, which in turn disperse the moisture to the skin. As a Water point, SP9 can be particularly useful in reducing swelling and oedema. This channel opens at the mouth and, when healthy, the lips will be red and moist: The 'Spleen's brilliance is manifested in the lips' (Su Wen in Kaptchuk 1983, p.59).

GALL BLADDER 41 ZU LIN QI (FOOT ABOVE TEARS)

Location: In the depression distal to the junction of the fourth and fifth metatarsals on the lateral side of the extensor digiti minimi tendon.

Element: Wood.

Functions: Spreads stagnant Liver Qi, clears Fire and extinguishes Wind, clears vision and sharpens hearing.

Applications: Eye diseases, eye redness and swelling, headache and vertigo.

Gall Bladder 41 (GB41) is a Shu-Stream point, which is where the Qi pours through the channel. GB41 is used in a Facial Enhancement Acupuncture treatment purely for its benefit of helping the eyes. This is a great point for clarity when the eyes appear cloudy or unfocused.

STOMACH 44 NEI TING (INNER COURTYARD)

Location: Between the second and third toes at the edge of the interdigital skin at the dividing line between red and white flesh.

Element: Earth.

Functions: Regulates and harmonises the Stomach and intestines, regulates Qi and stops pain.

Applications: Dysfunctions of the five sensory organs (e.g. toothache), peripheral facial paralysis, frontal headache and stomach pain.

Stomach 44 (ST44) is a Ying Spring point, where the Qi trickles down the meridian. A very important use of ST44, in the context of a Facial Enhancement Acupuncture treatment, is its ability to improve the complexion. It is 'indicated for heat disorders affecting the upper portion of the channel in the face and head as well as clearing heat and damp-heat from the intestines' (Deadman 1993, p.34). When used in conjunction with Large Intestine 4 (LI4), ST44 can help to expel Wind from the face.

By using GB41 and ST44 on the feet, we are also aiming to ground the Qi, whilst so much attention is given to the face and head.

3.3 ACUPUNCTURE POINTS ON THE HANDS AND ARMS

Acupuncture anaesthesia is a subject that fascinates me and, during the Facial Enhancement Acupuncture treatment, we employ a few anaesthetic points on the hands and arms to help patients with the needle experience. Most patients who have a FEA treatment do not find the needles to be too much of a problem at all; however, I have found that patients are a lot more comfortable when anaesthetic points are used during the session.

Various studies have been written about acupuncture as an anaesthetic and what has been published makes for very interesting reading. Much of the research that influenced this aspect of my protocol was documented in the 1970s, which we will come to later. However, I have also chosen to highlight some studies in the 1990s, which have continued to provide evidence of the benefits of using acupuncture for anaesthesia. The first two research papers demonstrate how electroacupuncture (EA) is being used for this purpose.

In 1996, 59 patients were split into two groups to undergo a colonoscopy with either electroacupuncture analgesia or meperidine analgesia. Meperidine is an opioid drug commonly used for this type of procedure. The acupuncture points used in the study were ST36 and Stomach 37 (ST37) on the right, and the auricular point Shen Men on both sides. The needles were inserted ten minutes before and retained throughout the colonoscopic examination. The conclusion was that 'the analgesic effect of elecroacupuncture and meperidine is the same but EA has fewer side-effects' (Wang *et al.* 1996, pp.13–20).

Another study, published in 1999, compared the results of electroacupuncture to the pharmacological product alfentanil during oocyte aspiration for in-vitro fertilisation. Both the acupuncture and alfentanil were combined with a paracervical block (PCB). LI4, Triple Heater 5 (TH5), Stomach 29 (ST29), Du Mai 20 (DU20) and ST36 were attached to EA and others with manual stimulation:

> In conclusion, this study has shown that EA is as good an anaesthetic method as alfentanil during oocyte aspiration. The women in this study were positive to the idea of using EA. We therefore suggest that EA may be a good alternative to conventional anaesthesia during oocyte aspiration. (Stener-Victorin *et al.* 1999, p.2483)

Finally, a 1992 study compared acupuncture at ST36 and LI4 to epidural anaesthesia in appendectomy. Eighty patients with appendicitis were divided equally, with one group receiving epidural anaesthesia and the other receiving acupuncture only. Both groups performed well during the surgery; however, what was interesting was that the acupuncture group fared better in terms of associated signs:

> There were less respiratory depression, hypotension, cardiac arrhythmia and less amount of liquid infusion needed than

that of the epidural block during operation. Furthermore, in the group of acupuncture anesthesia, the intestinal gas excreted earlier, the analgetics and antibiotics administered were less and the rate of the wound infection were reduced after operation. (Sun, Li and Si 1992, pp.87–89)

LI4 forms part of the Facial Enhancement Acupuncture protocol, in part for its use as an analgesic. According to *Acupuncture Anesthesia*, LI4 is 'used in all types of acupuncture anesthesia surgery' and 'the area for pain relieving is very strong' (Anon. 1975, p.202).

I selected two other points on the arm, based on their documented anaesthetic effects: Triple Heater 8 (TH8) and Pericardium 4 (PC4). I first read about the use of these points for lung surgery in *The Principles and Practical Use of Acupuncture Anaesthesia* (Anon. 1974), whilst studying, and the discovery made a big impression. What astounded me was that, in the 1960s, doctors and surgeons of the Peking Tuberculosis Research Institute had managed to reduce the 40 needles, used for anaesthesia to remove parts of the lung, to only one. This single needle was used to deeply penetrate the arm in order to stimulate both TH8 and PC4: 'Two hundred and one of the operations were performed with anaesthesia from a single needle, and 98.5 percent of these were successful' (Anon. 1974, p.277). Practitioners found that TH8 'is highly effective in nullifying pain' and PC4 'functions like a sedative' (Anon. 1974, p.279). This was witnessed in 1974 by ten Canadian anaesthetists who visited China to view acupuncture analgesia first-hand: 'The most dramatic exposition was the use of a single needle, stimulating San-Yin-Loh (TB-8) and Hsi-men (EH-4), and providing analgesia for thoracotomy' (Spoerel 1975, p.363).

During Facial Enhancement Acupuncture, we are obviously not performing anything near as invasive as opening the chest cavity; these points are particularly relevant to this type of surgery due to the region of the meridians. Nor are we, you will no doubt be relieved to hear, needling through the arm. However, we are using these points for their general analgesic and sedation effects and because they may help to 'calm the heart and secure the spirit' (Anon. 1975, p.198).

Acupuncture anaesthesia is a vast subject and if, like me, you find this subject of particular interest, more of the research can be found in my first book, *The Pocket Guide to Facial Enhancement Acupuncture* (Adkins 2006).

However, all of these studies serve to demonstrate that if acupuncture can achieve such a response as to provide pain-free procedures such as these, imagine what can be done by using similar points in a Facial Enhancement treatment. There should be no reason why anyone should experience any discomfort during a FEA session.

The points on the hands and arms that I have chosen for their analgesic effects follow. As you can see from the studies I have selected, aside from LI4, which I would always recommend, this list is not exclusive for analgesia but, in my experience, these points have always benefited the patient during treatment. Other points that can also be utilised for this purpose will be covered in the section dedicated to auricular points in Section 3.10.

LARGE INTESTINE 4 HE GU (JOINING THE VALLEY)

Location: In the webbing of the thumb and index finger at the highest spot of the muscle when the thumb and index finger are brought together.

Element: Metal.

Functions: The point for all facial symptoms, disperses wind and suppresses pain.

Applications: Can reduce headache pain, toothache, shoulder pain and also alleviates pain and inflammation of the hand, wrist, elbow, shoulder and neck.

LI4, in combination with LV3, is a famous ancient formula called the 'Four Gates' and is used for alleviating pain and stress. It is a very powerful method and balances the body's Qi, opening circulation throughout the meridians. Like LV3, LI4 is also a Source point and is indicated for many conditions. When needled, LI4 often produces a strong sensation or ache.

The Large Intestine meridian travels up to the face, so almost any symptom related to that region calls for this point. There is evidence that by needling LI4 in healthy volunteers, the blood perfusion volume of the bilateral acupuncture areas of the face are effectively increased (Wang *et al.* 2012). Studies such as this demonstrate why LI4 is such an important point in the Facial Enhancement Acupuncture protocol.

TRIPLE HEATER 8 SANYANGLUO
(THREE YANG CONNECTION)

Location: On the dorsal plane of the forearm, 4 cun above the transverse wrist crease, between the ulna and radius.

Element: Fire.

Functions: Needled through to PC4 in acupuncture anaesthesia, eases pain and removes blockages.

Applications: Toothache, voice loss, deafness, hand and arm pain.

As outlined in the section on acupuncture anaesthesia, Triple Heater 8 (TH8) is used in conjunction with PC4 as an anaesthetic point.

PERICARDIUM 4 XI MEN, HSIMAM
(GATE OF QI RESERVE)

Location: Between the *palmaris longus* and *flexor carpi radialis*, on the link line between Pericardium 3 (PC3) and Pericardium 7 (PC7), on the inside of the arm 5 cun above the transverse crease of the wrist.

Element: Fire.

Functions: Needled through the arm from TH8 in acupuncture anaesthesia, alleviates pain, clears heat from the Qi and calms the *Shen*.

Applications: Stops vomiting, heart pain, palpitations, coughing blood, pain of the elbow and arm.

PC4 is used as an analgesic point with TH8. Known as an Accumulation or Xi-Cleft point, PC4 is where Qi and Blood gather.

3.4 ACUPUNCTURE POINTS ON
THE HEAD AND FOREHEAD
DU MAI (GOVERNOR VESSEL) 20
BAI HUI (ONE HUNDRED MEETINGS)

Location: On the dorsal midline, 5 cun posterior to the anterior hairline on the crown of the head.

Functions: Calms the Spirit, soothes the Liver, raises Yang, benefits the head and counters prolapse.

Applications: Headache, heaviness of head, dizziness, tinnitus, nosebleed, poor memory and lockjaw.

The Du Mai channel is often translated as the Governor Vessel and DU20 is the highest acupuncture point on the body. I have heard this point referred to as 'Upright Pillar': a point where a patient would hang from a golden thread, which would keep them upright when they have the weight of the world on their shoulders. We are using DU20 in the context of a Facial Enhancement treatment to lift the face and to also relax the patient.

YINTANG (HALL OF IMPRESSION)

Location: Midpoint between the medial end of the eyebrows. See Figure 3.1.

Muscle: *Procerus.*

Functions: Calms the Spirit.

Applications: Frontal headache, sinus and eye issues and insomnia.

Yin Tang is an Extraordinary (Extra) point but, unlike other Extra points, it is found on the Du Mai channel. Many people describe its location as being in the region of the 'third eye'.

   As one of my favourite points to use for many treatments in the clinic, Yin Tang has a noticeable calming and relaxing effect on the patient. I have often likened it to closing the open windows on a computer screen, as the often busy mind of the patient quickly starts to shut down. Using this point towards the beginning of the facial acupuncture treatment is an effective preparation for the rest of the needling. It also activates the *procerus* muscle, opening up the area between the eyebrows.

BLADDER 6 CHENG GUANG (LIGHT GUARD)

Location: 1.5 cun lateral to the midline, 2.5 cun within the anterior hairline. See Figure 3.1.

Element: Water.

Functions: Enhances eyesight, alleviates pain, clears the head and eliminates wind.

Applications: Headache, glaucoma and dizziness.

Bladder 6 (BL6) is a point that is rarely used as its main functions are to clear the eyes.

In a Facial Enhancement Acupuncture session, we use BL6 purely for its location, although, when looking at anti-ageing as a whole, enhanced eyesight is a particularly good side-effect from using this point.

GALL BLADDER 14 YANGBAI (YANG WHITE)

Location: 1 cun above the eyebrow, directly in line with the pupil. See Figure 3.1.

Muscle: *Frontalis.*

Element: Wood.

Functions: Alleviates pain, enhances eyesight, expels wind and benefits the head.

Applications: Eye disease, headaches, facial paralysis, vertigo, drooping of the eyelid and deviation of the mouth.

Gall Bladder 14 (GB14) is a very good point for pain of the head and to benefit the eyes, in particular for sagging eyelids. It can also be used in cases of facial paralysis and has been chosen in many studies researching the treatment of Bell's Palsy using acupuncture: 'Bell's palsy is an acute peripheral unilateral facial weakness or paralysis with an as yet unknown cause' (Xia *et al.* 2011, p.1). At the time of writing, a study has just been published highlighting the positive effect of *De-Qi* for patients with early-onset Bell's Palsy: 'De Qi is an internal compound sensation of soreness, tingling, fullness, aching, cool, warmth and heaviness, and a radiating sensation at and around the acupoints' (Xu *et al.* 2013, p.1). Points included GB14, ST4, Stomach 6 (ST6), Stomach 7 (ST7) and Triple Heater 17 (TH17) on the affected side and LI4 on both sides. Six months following treatment, it was found that acupuncture with *De-Qi* 'improved facial muscle recovery, disability and quality of life among patients with Bell palsy. Stronger intensity of *De-Qi* was associated with better therapeutic effects' (Xu *et al.* 2013, p.5).

These recent findings are encouraging for the specific treatment of Bell's Palsy and for facial acupuncture in general, especially as half of these points are used in the Facial Enhancement Acupuncture protocol. Up until now, I have mainly limited *De-Qi* to the body points as, due to the many facial points involved, there was a potential for the treatment to be overwhelming if all points were needled in this way. A proportion of the points used have also been selected, in the most part, for their location and work with the underlying muscle group. To a certain extent, I will be aiming to achieve *De-Qi* for related points depending on the requirements of the patient and the specific facial issue they are looking for me to work upon. However, in light of this new research, I will certainly explore this in even more depth. It is important to remember that any protocol is organic and must continue to grow and develop for optimum results to be achieved. Despite Facial Enhancement Acupuncture already garnering effective results in my practice and for those trained in the protocol, acupuncture is a life-long study. I look forward to continuing to maximise the results of the treatment and reporting my findings in future publications.

Returning to GB14, the many studies for facial paralysis utilising this point unilaterally demonstrate its use for lifting the facial muscles. This is what we are aiming to achieve when using GB14, as it is located on the *frontalis* muscle, which is responsible for lifting the eyebrow. The method for needling GB14 outlined in Chapter 4 will demonstrate this muscle training technique.

FOREHEAD POINT

This is an additional point that I use in the protocol. Located approximately 1.5 cun (2.5cm) above Yin Tang, this point is used for reducing forehead tension, as well as lines and wrinkles in that area. See Figure 3.1.

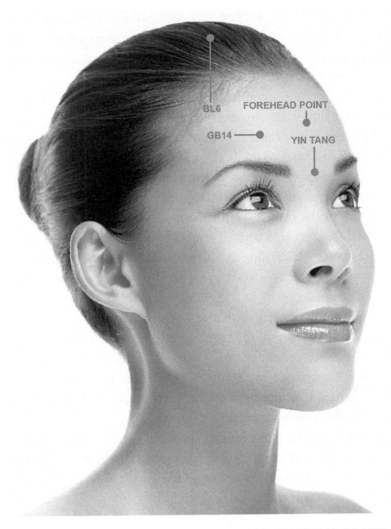

FIGURE 3.1 THE LOCATION OF THE HEAD AND FOREHEAD POINTS

3.5 ACUPUNCTURE POINTS AROUND THE EYES
BLADDER 2 ZAN SHU (COLLECT BAMBOO)

Location: In the depression at the medial end of the eyebrow. See Figure 3.2.

Muscle: *Frontalis* and *corrugator supercilli.*

Element: Water.

Functions: Clears heat, eliminates wind, enhances eyesight and alleviates pain.

Applications: Eye diseases, sinusitis, headache, neck pain and stiffness.

Bladder 2 (BL2) is a really good point for benefiting the eyes and also the sinuses; we are using it predominantly as a lifting point to raise the medial end of the eyebrow. The underlying muscle is the *corrugator supercilli*, which is responsible for the vertical frown lines on the forehead. Targeting this point helps to tighten the muscle to prevent these lines from forming.

YUYAO (FISH WAIST)

Location: Directly above the pupil in the eyebrow. See Figure 3.2.

Muscle: At the top of the *orbicularis oculi*, where it meets the *frontalis*.

Functions: Enhances eyesight, activates the vessels, relaxes tendons and reduces oedema.

Applications: Oculomotor paresis, eye tics and eye disease.

Yuyao is an Extra point that is located in the middle of the eyebrow. We are using this point to help raise this area. Interestingly, Yuyao was reported by the Shanghai First College of Medicine as an anaesthetic point for use in minor surgery to the forehead, eyebrow and temple regions (Anon. 1975). This can only serve to continue to lessen any discomfort that may otherwise be felt when we work more closely on these parts of the face.

TRIPLE HEATER 23 ZHU KONG (SILK BAMBOO HOLLOW)

Location: The lateral end of the eyebrow, in the depression on the supraorbital margin. See Figure 3.2.

Muscle: *Orbicularis oculi*.

Element: Fire.

Functions: Enhances eyesight, alleviates pain, expels wind and clears heat.

Applications: Eye diseases, eye tics, one-sided headache, toothache, deviation of the face and eye.

Triple Heater 23 (TH23) is another acupuncture point that can be used to benefit the eyes. Here, we are using this point to lift the lateral end of the eyebrow and raise drooping eyelids.

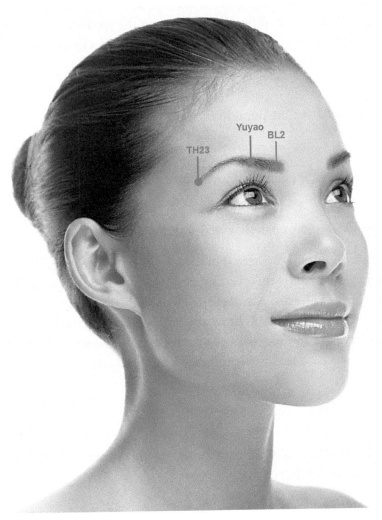

FIGURE 3.2 THE LOCATION OF THE POINTS USED AROUND THE EYES

3.6 ACUPUNCTURE POINTS ON THE JAW
JAW POINTS

These are six Extra points that I use on either side of the mandible to tighten the jaw line.

Location: Find Stomach 5 (ST5) Da Ying (Great Welcome), which is 1.3 cun anterior and inferior to the corner of the jaw, on the front edge of the *masseter* muscle. The first point is directly below ST5, with one point approximately 1.5 cun either side. See Figure 3.3.

Muscle: *Platysma.*

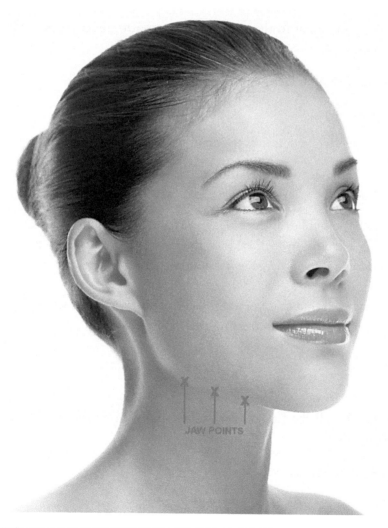

FIGURE 3.3 THE POSITIONING OF THE JAW POINTS

3.7 ACUPUNCTURE POINTS ON THE FRONT OF THE FACE

CHEEK POINT

This is another Extra point that I have chosen for its capacity to tighten the cheek area.

Location: Approximately 1–2 cun above ST5, then 1 cun back towards the ear and into the cheek muscle. See Figure 3.4.

Muscle: *Masseter.*

STOMACH 4 DICANG (EARTH GRANARY)

Location: 0.4 cun lateral to the corner of the mouth, directly below the pupil. See Figure 3.4.

Muscle: *Orbicularis oris, risorius* and *zygomaticus major.*

Element: Earth.

Functions: Expels wind, activates the channel and alleviates pain.

Applications: Facial paralysis, deviation of the mouth, toothache, neuralgia and night blindness.

Stomach 4 (ST4) often lies at the base of the nasal labial fold. We are using ST4 purely for its location at the side of the mouth as we are angling it up into the underlying *zygomaticus major* muscle, responsible for raising the smile.

ST4 is also a common point used for facial paralysis and was selected for the aforementioned study into treating Bell's Palsy.

LARGE INTESTINE 20 LINGXIANG (WELCOME FRAGRANCE)

Location: Level with the lateral part of the nasal wing in the nasal labial fold. See Figure 3.4.

Muscle: *Levator labii superioris.*

Element: Metal.

Functions: Opens the nasal passages, expels wind and clears heat.

Applications: Deviation of the mouth, facial paralysis, rhinitis, nosebleed, facial oedema and facial itching.

Large Intestine 20 (LI20) is a local point for swelling, paralysis and itching of the face. The point is located at the top of the nasal labial fold, which covers the *levator labii superioris* muscle. Points along the Large Intestine channel are used to detoxify and improve the complexion.

STOMACH 3 JU LIAO (GREAT CHEEKBONE)

Location: Directly below the pupil on the lower border of the ala nasi. See Figure 3.4.

Muscle: *Levator labii superioris* and *levator angular oris*.

Element: Earth.

Functions: Enhances eyesight, expels wind and activates the channel.

Applications: Mouth and eye deviation, sinus pain, swelling of the lips and cheeks and facial paralysis.

This point is used in conjunction with LI20 and Small Intestine 18 (SI18) to shape and contour the cheek area. The *levator angular oris* is a muscle that underlies the *levator labii superioris* and this is triggered when needling, helping to lift the face.

SMALL INTESTINE 18 QUANLIAO (CHEEKBONE CREVICE)

Location: In the depression below the zygomatic bone, directly below the outer canthus. See Figure 3.4.

Muscle: *Zygomaticus major*.

Element: Fire.

Functions: Alleviates pain, activates the channel, returns to correct position and relieves cramp, expels wind and reduces swelling.

Applications: Facial paralysis, facial cramps, deviation of the mouth and eye, facial pain and toothache.

Small Intestine 18 (SI18) is used in conjunction with ST3 and LI20. Aside from its outlined functions and applications, needling this point has an effect on the *zygomaticus major* muscle in order to lift the face.

STOMACH 2 SI BAI (FOUR WHITES)

Location: In the depression of the infraorbital foramen, 1 cun directly below the pupil. See Figure 3.4.

Muscle: *Orbicularis oculi.*

Element: Earth.

Functions: Enhances eyesight, clears heat and expels wind.

Applications: Eye diseases, headache, night blindness and deviation of the mouth and eye.

Stomach 2 (ST2) is located on the *orbicularis oculi* muscle. Locate the point, gently press your finger to it and tightly squeeze your eye shut. This muscle is responsible for closing your eyelid, but you will feel how the skin is drawn in around the eye and forehead. It is this action that gradually forms crow's feet around the eye. We needle this point to lift the top of the cheek and to benefit the eyes.

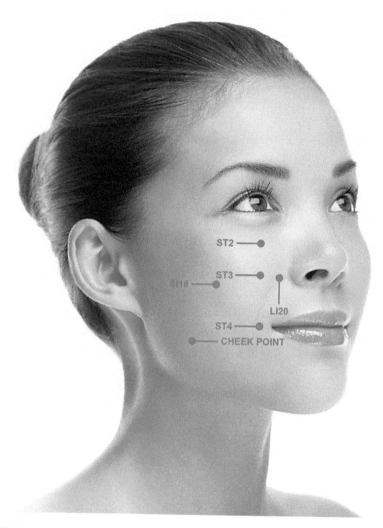

FIGURE 3.4 THE LOCATION OF THE POINTS USED
ON THE FRONT OF THE FACE

3.8 ACUPUNCTURE POINT ON THE CHIN
REN MAI (CONCEPTION VESSEL) 24
CHENG JIANG (RECEIVING FLUID)

Location: Below the middle of the lower lip, in the depression of the mentolabial fold. See Figure 3.5.

Muscle: Between *orbicularis oris* and *mentalis*.

Functions: Reduces oedema, alleviates pain, activates the channel and its vessels, benefits the face, clears heat, calms the Spirit and expels wind.

Applications: Deviation of the mouth and eye, purple lips, swelling of the face, dry mouth, sweating, facial pareses and acute toothache.

According to the famed Chinese physician Li Shi Zhen, the Ren channel 'became the ocean or controller of the yin meridians' and at Ren 24 it meets with 'the du mai, large intestine and stomach meridians; then circles around the lips on the inside of the mouth, divides and passes up to chenqi [ST-1] where it ends' (Li Shi Zhen 1570 in Matsumoto and Birch 1986, pp.27–28). This demonstrates how needling this point can have a beneficial effect on the front of the face. It is also the only Yin point on the whole of the face, which could indicate its function to cool things down.

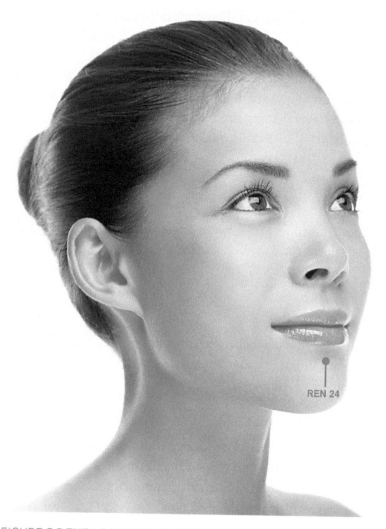

FIGURE 3.5 THE LOCATION OF REN 24

3.9 ACUPUNCTURE POINTS TO TREAT THE NECK

When treating the neck using Facial Enhancement Acupuncture, there are a few conditions that you can address using your acupuncture needles. Patients will ask you if it is possible to help with the sagging muscles in the neck. Some will refer to it as a 'turkey neck', which to my mind is not a nice description.

What you will find, as you work with more patients, is that the neck area is the place that starts to show ageing more than many others. When you look at the celebrities who have had thousands of pounds' worth of plastic surgery carried out, it is very often the neck that gives the game away. The points that I have outlined will all help to tighten the neck muscles and improve the overall appearance of this area. If the patient has a lot of lines around the neck, which may also extend down to the upper chest area, then this might be a candidate for using the dermal roller or dermal pen that we will explore in more detail in Section 5.3.

SMALL INTESTINE 17 TIAN RONG (HEAVENLY APPEARANCE)

Location: In the depression between the angle of the mandible and the anterior border of the *sternocleidomastoid*. See Figure 3.6.

Muscle: *Sternocleidomastoid.*

Element: Fire.

Functions: Reduces oedema, enhances hearing, descends rebellious Qi and benefits the neck and throat.

Applications: Tinnitus, deafness, acute throat inflammation, asthma, goitre and asthma.

Small Intestine 17 (SI17) helps to reduce swelling in the region of the neck. Deadman and Al-Khafaji also suggest that it can be used for swelling of the cheek (1993, p.34). In Five Element Acupuncture, SI17 is known as a 'Window of the Sky' point. This is a point that many regard as one of a selection of ten that have a connection with the Mind and Spirit of a patient. Therefore, it should help to balance and calm everything down. The translated name 'Heavenly Appearance' certainly seems quite apt for what we are trying to achieve. In the context of a Facial Enhancement Acupuncture treatment, we are using it to tighten the neck.

TRIPLE HEATER 17 YI FENG (WIND SCREEN)

Location: In the depression between the mastoid process and the mandible, behind the earlobe. See Figure 3.6.

Muscle: *Sternocleidomastoid.*

Triple Heater 17 (TH17) is not used directly in the treatment; it is listed here for its location. The Step-by-Step Guide in Chapter 4 will demonstrate how we needle up to this point from SI17.

REN MAI (CONCEPTION VESSEL) 23 LIAN QUAN (ANGLE SPRING)

Location: In the depression superior to the hyoid bone, on the ventral midline. See Figure 3.6.

Functions: Descends Qi, benefits the tongue and alleviates cough.

Applications: Throat disorders, mouth ulcers, lockjaw and dryness of the mouth.

Ren 23 is a central point on the neck and targets the *suprahyoid* muscles. Working with this point is part of the tightening and lifting process we are aiming to achieve in this area.

STOMACH 9 RENYING (PEOPLE WELCOME)

Location: 1.5 cun lateral to the upper side of the laryngeal prominence, on the front side of the *sternocleidomastoid* muscle. See Figure 3.6.

Muscle: *Sternocleidomastoid.*

Element: Earth.

Functions: Regulates Qi, alleviates pain, clears heat and benefits the throat and neck.

Applications: Asthma, hypertension, hypotension, throat inflammation and swelling, tonsillitis, headache.

Stomach 9 (ST9) is a very interesting point and warrants an in-depth look at how powerful a point it can be. Like SI17, in Five Element Acupuncture, ST9 is known as a 'Window of the Sky' point.

I have always considered ST9 to be a highly important point to use in a Facial Enhancement Acupuncture treatment, not simply because of its location on the neck, but also because of its power to open up the face and improve the complexion. This is very clearly highlighted by Wei Lushang and Xiao Fei in their article for the *Journal of Chinese Medicine* in May 1997. It was noted that in using ST9 for patients with facial paralysis, as well as improvements to the paralysis, there was also a dramatic enhancement to their complexions and the smoothness of the skin's surface. Their research also showed that patients who suffered with problematic cerebral blood supply found that their 'complexions became lustrous and their eyes brightened' (Lushang and Fei 1997, p.18).

Doctors Wei Lushang and Xiao Fei also made studies into the effects of needling ST9 to improve particular skin conditions. Their results were quite astounding. In the case of chloasma, which is typified by a discolouring of the facial skin – for example, yellowish brown or coffee coloured patches – there were very dramatic reductions in its appearance after a few treatments. And, in some cases the condition completely cleared after a course of ten sessions using ST9 (Lushang and Fei 2007).

Another complaint that I am asked about frequently is acne and how acupuncture can help. Acne is a condition caused by over-secretion of the sebaceous glands, which can block the pores and cause break-outs (see Section 6.5). Needling ST9 on a regular basis has been found to be fairly effective in restricting the production of the sebaceous glands and has improved the acne over a course of treatments (Lushang and Fei 2007).

Generally, it has become apparent to me that ST9 is one of the most powerful acupuncture points at our disposal, which may be why we are often instructed to use it with caution. However, due to its many benefits, I feel that it is a point that we should consider using more frequently.

STOMACH 13 QI HU (QI DOOR)

Location: 4 cun lateral to the midline, at the top of the chest directly beneath Stomach 12 (ST12) and the lower side of the clavical. See Figure 3.6.

Element: Earth.

Functions: Unbinds the chest, relieves breathing problems and descends rebellious Qi.

Applications: Pain in the chest, asthma, wheezing, stiffness of the neck and vomiting blood.

Stomach 13 (ST13) and the following point, Gall Bladder 21 (GB21), are to be viewed as optional additions, as not all patients will require treatment on their necks. ST13 is a point used for treating the lungs; if the lungs are working freely, tension to the neck muscles will be reduced.

Note: Needle with extreme caution as deep insertion carries a substantial risk of lung puncture.

GALL BLADDER 21 JIAN JING (SHOULDER WELL)

Location: On the high point of the *trapezius* muscle, at the point of greatest tenderness. See Figure 3.6.

Element: Wood.

Functions: Alleviates pain, regulates Qi, activates the channel, clears heat and expels wind.

Applications: Neck pain and stiffness, shoulder and back pain, breast pain and prolonged labour.

GB21 is located on the high point of the *trapezius* muscle, and is a powerful valve for unblocking energy. When the smooth flow of energy is achieved in this area, the neck becomes less tense and Qi flows freely:

> So strong is the action of Jiangjing GB-21 in descending qi that Gao Wu, in the *Ode of Xi-hong*, says 'When you needle Jiangjing GB-21 you must needle Zusanli ST-36. If this is not done, the qi will not be regulated.' (Deadman, Al-Khafaji and Baker 2001, p.439).

ST36 forms part of the Facial Enhancement Acupuncture protocol and Gao Wu's words demonstrate the benefit of needling the feet and legs, before beginning work on the face and upper body in this treatment.

Note: Contraindicated in pregnancy.

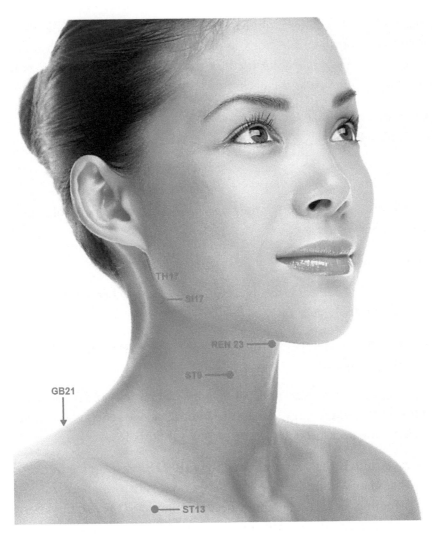

FIGURE 3.6 THE LOCATION OF THE POINTS USED ON THE NECK

3.10 AURICULAR ACUPUNCTURE POINTS FOR FACIAL ENHANCEMENT ACUPUNCTURE

Auricular acupuncture, or ear acupuncture as it is also known, uses similar skills to traditional acupuncture, but with acupuncture stimulation limited to the external ear. When I studied Five Element Acupuncture, we did not cover any auricular practice in our studies; most of my research has been undertaken over the last few years. Since then I have discovered some very powerful treatments using points on the ear.

Traditional acupuncture has been practised for over 2500 years, at least, and ear acupuncture is thought to have been around for the same length of time, albeit without the same notoriety. Auricular therapy has a long history of use in China. It was mentioned in the most famous of ancient Chinese medical textbooks, the *Nei Jing*: 'This ancient Chinese document was very specific about the needling of particular auricular points for the balancing of functional disorders related to a particular channel system' (Ken and Yongqiang 1991).

Auricular acupuncture owes a lot of its current popularity to the late Dr Paul Nogier, a French physician from Lyon. He is credited for research and development of auricular acupuncture since the 1950s and has even been nicknamed the 'Father of modern auricolotherapy' by the Chinese (Gori and Firenzuoli 2007, p.14). He famously 'drew a chart of ear points that was mapped from the shape of an inverted fetus' (Chen 2004, p.3). This microsystem meant that by stimulating points on the ear, the whole body could be treated.

Following on from this concept, we can look at various auricular points that will have some bearing on our Facial Enhancement Acupuncture treatment. Many acupuncturists who I know and have worked with are not that familiar with the points of the ear, unless of course they are auricular specialists. These points are some of the most powerful and many practitioners achieve fantastic results with their patients by only using these points. In fact, there are many successful acupuncturists who run only auricular clinics. There are several fine publications specialising in auricular acupuncture and they all seem to feature very accurate diagrams showing the many points on the ear. It may be worth purchasing a large Nogier wall chart for your clinic; this will give you an instant reference when deciding which point you should choose.

Personally, I will always use the point Shen Men left, then right for every FEA treatment that I perform. It is an effective point to use in combination with classical points like Yin Tang and DU20 for relaxation and calming. Also, in conjunction with this, I will choose to use another auricular point that would correspond with a particular area of the face that I am keen to work on. For example, if I am interested in improving the area around the eyes, then I might consider auricular points that relate to this.

Some of the points that I have found to be most successful, alongside Shen Men, are the points Mandible, Eyes, Cheek and Mouth. However, you will be able to use the initial consultation to gauge which area to focus on for each particular patient. My advice for any auricular points would be to research them and see what points work for you and then incorporate them into your own treatment protocol.

When needling auricular points I like to use a 15mm (length) × 0,20mm (thickness)/36 (gauge) needle, I find it advisable to use a sterile swab to clean the ear prior to this. This area can be very vulnerable and must be scrupulously clean before you begin.

Listed below are a few auricular points that could work well in a Facial Enhancement Acupuncture treatment. See Figure 3.7.

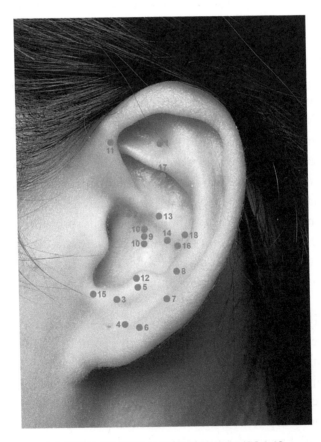

FIGURE 3.7 THE LOCATION OF THE AURICULAR POINTS 1–18

1. SHEN MEN

Like its counterpart on the body, Shen Men is a powerful point for calming the Spirit. It can also be used as an analgesic in combination with the three constitutional anaesthetic points. It should be needled first, before selecting a follow-up point.

2. MOUTH

Relates to mouth issues (e.g. cold sores).

3. FOREHEAD

This point is often used for headaches, but in this context can be employed for enhancing the forehead.

4. EYE

Can be used for improving vision and brightening the eyes.

5. TEMPLE

As you can guess, Temple is used specifically for headaches in this location. However, it can also be used to focus on this area of the face.

6. CHEEK

This point is also known as Face and is used for cases of facial paralysis and working with the facial muscles. It is recommended for treatment involving this part of the face, so it would be a useful point to include, particularly for lifting the cheek.

7. MANDIBLE

Also known as Jaw, this can be selected to target jowls.

8. NECK

Again, relating directly to its name, this point can be used to relieve tension in the neck.

9. HEART

This point has some correlation with Shen Men.

10. LUNG

As the Lung governs the skin, either Lung 1 (LU1) or Lung 2 (LU2) can be used to improve the complexion. Anyone presenting with skin rashes, rosacea or acne could benefit from this auricular point.

11. SYMPATHETIC

This is a pain-relieving point, so it would combine nicely with LI4, PC4 and TH8.

12. SUBCORTEX

This point is known for its anti-inflammatory effects and can reduce swelling. Therefore, it will help the face to calm down during the treatment. It is also a point used for acupuncture analgesia, so it would work well with the anaesthetic points and boost the effects.

13. ZERO POINT

'Zero Point is thought to have a powerful influence in treating various conditions including pain, sedation, addiction treatment, and inflammation' (Frank and Soliman 1999, p.13). This point is also deemed to bring the whole body back into balance, and this homeostasis will be beneficial not only for how your patient looks but for how they feel too.

14. RELAX MUSCLE

An auricular point that literally does what its name suggests and relaxes the patient's muscles. This can be beneficial for patients who are struggling to unwind and really enjoy the treatment.

15. ENDOCRINE

This system in our bodies is responsible for the secretion of hormones into our bloodstream. So, where skin issues are caused by hormonal imbalances, this point can be used help address this. Also, when the Endocrine system is working efficiently, it will slow down the ageing process and assist in retaining our vitality as we get older.

16. SPLEEN

In Section 3.2 we discussed how the Spleen sends fluid up to the lungs and they then disperse moisture in the skin, so this point can assist with hydration. Choosing the Spleen point on the ear can also help to tone the flesh, as discussed in Section 1.1.9.

17. KIDNEY

This organ relates to the ageing process as the Kidney governs all stages of development. If your patient has bluish eye bags, you may like to try this point as the Kidney is often linked to this problem.

18. LIVER

The Liver is linked to the eyes and we can use this point to directly improve this area and decrease dark circles.

CHAPTER 4

STEP-BY-STEP GUIDE TO THE FACIAL ENHANCEMENT ACUPUNCTURE PROTOCOL

4.1 CONTRAINDICATIONS

The training acupuncturists are given ensures that we take a thorough patient history before we commence treatment. This is also crucial when conducting a cosmetic acupuncture treatment and I provide a free 15-minute initial consultation to determine whether someone is able to undergo the procedure and to describe what they can expect from a course of Facial Enhancement Acupuncture.

The first thing to consider would be whether the patient has recently had more invasive cosmetic treatments such as microdermabrasion, laser resurfacing or a surgical facelift. I would also check to see if they have had recent Botox® or fillers. It would be possible to work on areas that have not been injected; however, I like to wait at least three months before carrying out Facial Enhancement Acupuncture in these cases.

From a health perspective, I would refrain from performing a cosmetic acupuncture treatment if a person suffers from chronic migraines, uncontrolled high blood pressure or diabetes, has cancer, is actively trying for a baby, pregnant or breast-feeding, has had a pacemaker fitted, during a cold or flu, during an allergic reaction or if someone has a problem with excessive bleeding or bruising.

Sometimes it is possible to treat the patient's current health problems and then re-evaluate them at a later date to establish if they are now able to receive Facial Enhancement Acupuncture.

As with any Five Element Acupuncture treatment, I am always conscious to look out for any indications that may need me to refer the patient to a medical practitioner and the same applies with my facial procedure. If at any time I am aware of the symptoms or conditions of an illness that cause me any concern, then I will always refer the patient to a medical consultant.

4.2 PREPARATION

Before you start your Facial Enhancement Acupuncture treatment, and even prior to your patient arriving at the clinic, make sure that you are well prepared and have your supplies ready. You will need cotton wool and cotton buds and also some cleanser to remove any make-up or just to cleanse your patient's face before you start the facial treatment. We will go into more depth in Step 4.3.4 of the treatment protocol, but it is recommended to have some skin-numbing cream and arnica on hand. Tweezers are also necessary for insertion of the intradermal needles.

Like any traditional acupuncture treatment, you will need to be able to access your patient's feet, legs, hands and arms, so that you can use the constitutional acupuncture points before you start working on the face. These points will be used to ground and relax the patient in order to make the treatment as pleasurable as possible.

The amount of time that you set aside for FEA treatment is entirely up to you and you will get this down to a fine art once you have carried out a few sessions. Personally, I like to allow at least two hours for my first treatment, as we will need to carry out an in-depth initial consultation and we will be adding in a clearing or detox protocol. Subsequently, my sessions are 75 minutes, but I allow an hour and a half, so that the patient has time to relax and not feel rushed following the treatment.

4.3 STEP-BY-STEP GUIDE TO FACIAL ENHANCEMENT ACUPUNCTURE
4.3.1 INITIAL GROUNDING TREATMENT

How we start a treatment is very much down to the preferences of the practitioner. Before we embark on a series of treatments it is important that we perform some sort of detox or clearing treatment on the patient. (This clearing treatment is usually only performed on the first visit.)

Because of my Five Element background and training, the obvious choice for me would be to perform an Aggressive Energy Drain on the patient. See Section 3.1 for more on this protocol.

BL13, BL14, BL15, BL18, BL20 and BL23

To begin, make sure that your patient is comfortable, as it can take some time for the AE to clear. You will need to insert the needles at the points listed bilaterally and very superficially. At this stage, do not needle BL15, the Heart Shu point; this point should be needled on its own after testing for AE on the other points. Also, remember that we need to use a couple of dummy needles that are inserted level with, or just outside of, the Bladder meridian, after the main Shu points have been needled. This ensures that the Shu points are correct, as the redness should be less pronounced at the control points.

This stage of treatment depends on how long the redness takes to completely clear or 'drain'.

The needles for the AE Drain should be retained until the erythema around the needles has cleared. If very little or no redness appears, then retain the needles for a few minutes and then remove.

I would encourage you to try to get into the routine of performing an AE Drain for the first treatment when you take on a new Facial Enhancement patient. If you feel things are not progressing very well during the course of facial treatments, it may be worth repeating the AE Drain to make sure all energy is clear. As a Five Element practitioner, I am very familiar with this type of treatment. However, depending on your background, you may wish to utilise your own protocol for draining AE, detoxing or clearing.

Remember to make your patient fully aware, during their initial consultation, that you will be using body points, as they may only expect facial treatment. Once any AE has been cleared from a patient, you should see a dramatic response to treatment and a vast improvement in their Mind, Body and Spirit. This will form the optimum basis for further treatment.

Again, depending on your school of acupuncture, I would take the patient's pulses and also investigate their general health condition before starting the treatments.

4.3.2 NEEDLING THE LEGS AND FEET
LV3, ST36, SP9, GB41 and ST44

These points provide an ideal base for the patient before we begin work on the face, they should be needled every treatment. I always start to needle the points on the patient's feet and legs first. These points are designed to give a good grounding for the treatment. They are retained throughout and are the last needles to be removed.

Needle size: 25mm (length) × 0,16mm (thickness)/40 (gauge).

Technique: Bilaterally and with slight tonification.

4.3.3 NEEDLING THE HANDS AND ARMS

This step utilises the anaesthetic nature of the selected points.

LI4, PC4 and TH8
Needle size: 25mm (length) × 0,16mm (thickness)/40 (gauge).

Technique: Bilaterally. It is important to achieve *De-Qi*. Always use LI4 as it forms part of the Four Gates treatment and has so many benefits. I mostly use PC4 and TH8 when a patient seems particularly nervous or jittery about the treatment and will benefit from extra sedation. These two points are situated on meridians that run into the chest area; this has a calming effect on the patient's respiration and helps them to relax during the procedure.

Note: LI4 is contraindicated in pregnancy.

4.3.4 NEEDLING THE HEAD AND FOREHEAD

Before we begin the facial needling, it is important to make sure that the skin is totally clean of any make-up and dirt. I would recommend a natural cleanser that does not contain chemicals.

If, despite using the points indicated for their anaesthetic properties, your patient is particularly sensitive to the facial needles, it might be worth considering the use of a mild anaesthetic cream. Lidocaine 5% can be applied to the areas of the face you will be paying particular attention to. This is similar to the cream that tattooists use in their studios. It needs to be applied at least 30 minutes prior to the facial needling and any residue should be removed before treatment commences. Use a disposable spatula, or similar tool, to apply the cream and try to avoid contact with your fingers at this stage, as much as possible. You can, of course, if you prefer, carry out the treatment without any cream; there is very little pain or discomfort due to the needles inserted during Section 4.3.3 and most of my treatments are done this way.

My needle preference has always been metal handles for traditional acupuncture. However, for facial work, I recommend plastic-handled needles as, due to their light weight, they remain more upright in the face, even with shallow needling. As the number of needles in use increases, the face is still accessible. This is helpful when we come to using the intradermals, as it will give you much more room to work on the face.

When conducting a Facial Enhancement Acupuncture treatment, it usually pays to stand or sit at the back of your patient, working over the top of their head and face. By needling from this position, you will always be using a lifting technique as you needle towards yourself. By continually using this technique, you will get into the habit of lifting the patient's face as you work.

DU20

Needle size: 25mm (length) × 0,16mm (thickness)/40 (gauge).

Technique: Evens.

Angle: 90 degrees perpendicular to the scalp.

Yin Tang

Use gentle stimulation upon insertion.

Needle size: 15mm (length) × 0,20mm (thickness)/36 (gauge).

Technique: Tonification.

Angle: Posterior, at approximately 75 degrees.

See Figure 4.1.

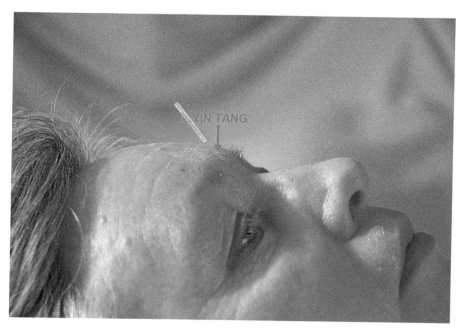

FIGURE 4.1 DEMONSTRATING NEEDLING AT YIN TANG

BL6

Needle size: 25mm (length) × 0,16mm (thickness)/40 (gauge).

Technique: This point is needled as you pull back on the patient's forehead. Pull the skin gently towards the rear of the head and then insert the needle. You are effectively pinning back the scalp using this method. Needle bilaterally, using evens technique.

Angle: Posterior, at approximately a 45-degree angle to the scalp.

See Figure 4.2.

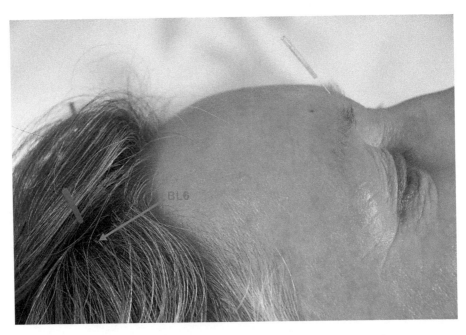

FIGURE 4.2 DEMONSTRATING NEEDLING IN THE HAIRLINE AT BL6

GB14

Needle size: 15mm (length) × 0,20mm (thickness)/36 (gauge).

Technique: When needling this point, do so bilaterally and use your other hand to pull back on the forehead. This will have the effect of pinning back the eyebrows. If you have needled this point correctly, the side that you have just needled will remain lifted when you take your other hand away. This is an effective combination with the intradermal needling you will carry out in Section 4.3.6 to raise the eyelids. Needle bilaterally, using evens technique.

Angle: Posterior and approximately 75 degrees from the forehead.

See Figure 4.3.

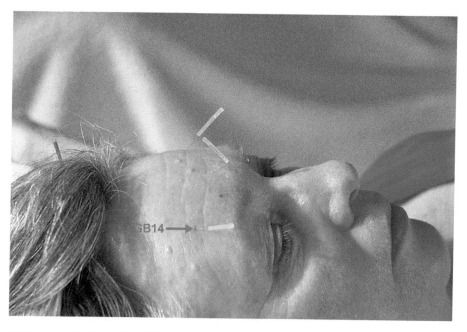

FIGURE 4.3 DEMONSTRATING NEEDLING AT GB14

Forehead Point

Needle size: 15mm (length) × 0,20mm (thickness)/36 (gauge).

Technique: Needle with an upwards motion.

See Figure 4.4.

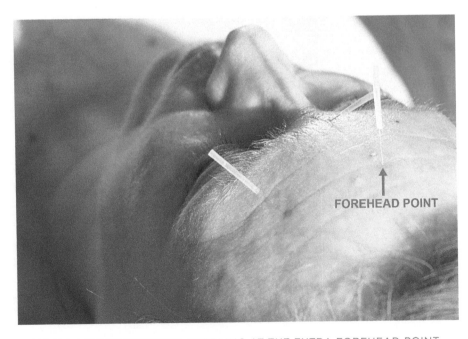

FIGURE 4.4 DEMONSTRATING NEEDLING AT THE EXTRA FOREHEAD POINT

4.3.5 NEEDLING THE EARS

At this stage of the Facial Enhancement Acupuncture treatment, we will also consider the use of some auricular points to support the treatment. I always include Shen Men, but you might also include points such as Mandible or Cheek. Your choice of ear points will be based on your initial consultation and will likely differ from patient to patient, depending on their requirements and your assessment. See Section 3.10 for details of auricular points that you may like to select. See Figure 4.5.

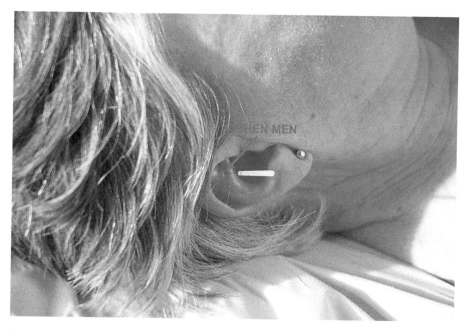

FIGURE 4.5 DEMONSTRATING NEEDLING AT THE AURICULAR POINT SHEN MEN

4.3.6 NEEDLING THE EYEBROW AREA

The next three points are needled using 6mm intradermals. It is best to insert them with tweezers. The type I recommend are those with a slanted tip and a wide handle grip. I find that these are the best to master this technique. By raising the eyebrows in this step, we will naturally lift the eyelids too. When needling any of the three eyebrow points, do not be afraid to lift the brow as much as possible; you need to be achieving a 'startled' look when you have finished inserting the needles.

Yuyao

Needle size: 6mm intradermal.

Technique: To needle this point, lift the eyebrow as you do so and pin it in place. This Extra point is one of the most sensitive points that you will needle on the face, so extra care needs to be taken when working in this area.

See Figure 4.6.

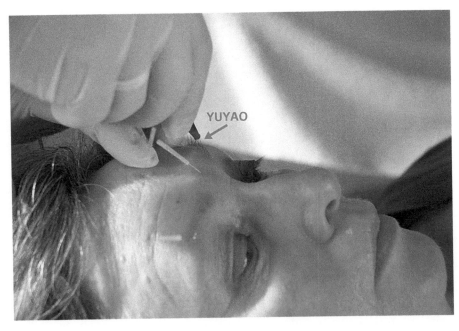

FIGURE 4.6 DEMONSTRATING NEEDLING AT YUYAO AND THE INTRADERMAL NEEDLING TECHNIQUE USING WIDE GRIP TWEEZERS

BL2

Needle size: 6mm intradermal.

Technique: Lift the medial end of the eyebrow with the forefinger of your other hand and needle with the intradermal, pinning the brow in an upward direction.

See Figure 4.7.

TH23

Needle size: 6mm intradermal.

Technique: TH23 this should be tackled in exactly the same way as the previous two points, again raising the brow as the intradermal needle is inserted.

See Figure 4.7.

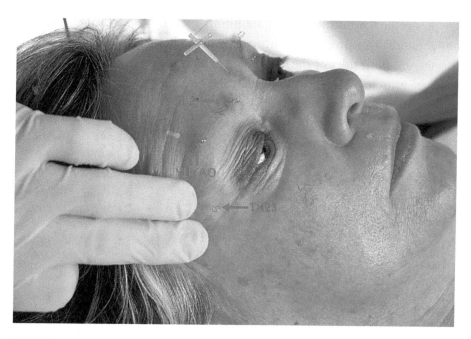

FIGURE 4.7 DEMONSTRATING THE EYEBROW NEEDLES IN PLACE

4.3.7 NEEDLING THE JAW

This technique is chiefly used for working on the patient's jowls. At this stage it might be worth mentioning needle technique. As a Classical Five Element practitioner, I was trained to needle without the use of guide tubes and, to date, this is my preferred needle technique. However, after years of carrying out facial treatments, it has become my experience that the whole treatment is less sensitive for the patient when using guide tubes for 25mm needling. This is particularly noticeable when treating the jowl area. I have found that patients find this technique more comfortable and it is easier to perform this next 'pinning' method.

Location: First, locate point ST5 and choose a point directly below it and one point symmetrically either side of this needle. Effectively, you will have three points under the mandible bone at approximately 1.5 cun distance between each point. These are not acupuncture points

Needle size: 25mm (length) × 0,16mm (thickness)/40 (gauge).

Technique: Apply downward pressure and tuck the skin under the jawbone as you needle the midpoint; you are pinning the flesh under the mandible bone. Repeat this procedure with the points either side. Needle the jaw in this way on both sides of the face. Over time, this part of the treatment will train the muscles in the jowl to tighten and encourage a more angular shape to the patient's jaw line.

See Figures 4.8 and 4.9.

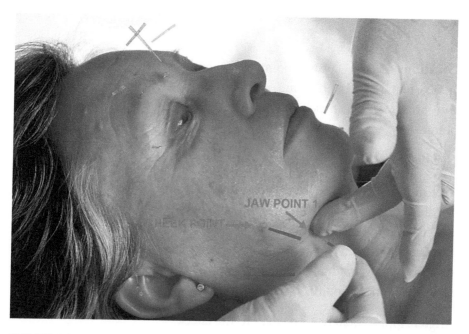

FIGURE 4.8 LOCATING THE FIRST JAW POINT AND TUCKING THE SKIN
BENEATH THE JAW BONE

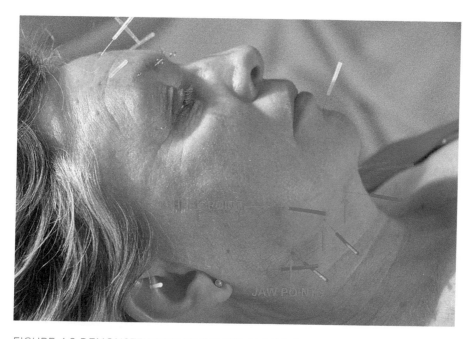

FIGURE 4.9 DEMONSTRATING NEEDLING ALONG THE JAW LINE

4.3.8 NEEDLING THE FRONT OF THE FACE
Cheek Point

Location: Again, locate point ST5 and palpate above this point approximately 1–2 cun in measurement, then 1 cun back towards the ear and into the cheek muscle. See Figures 4.8 and 4.9 for the location of the point.

Needle size: 25mm (length) × 0,16mm (thickness)/40 (gauge).

Technique: Needle this Extra point with insertion towards the ear. When needled correctly, there should be a 'grabbing' sensation as the needle enters the cheek muscle. If this is achieved, you will notice how the area we are working on tightens up almost immediately. This is a very important point that can give very dramatic results, so it is worth practising your needle techniques on this point. Needle bilaterally.

Angle: Approximately 45 degrees to the cheek.

See Figure 4.10.

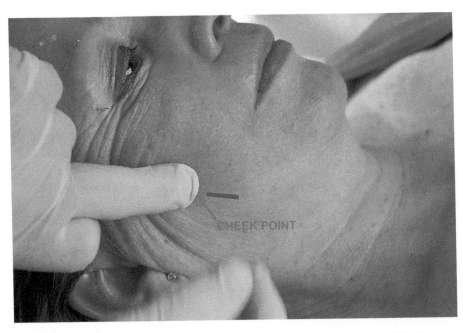

FIGURE 4.10 DEMONSTRATING HOW TO NEEDLE THE EXTRA CHEEK POINT

ST4

Needle size: 15mm (length) × 0,20mm (thickness)/36 (gauge).

Technique: Working with the 'smile' muscles and using the opposite hand to which you needle, pull up on the side of the mouth with your forefinger and insert a needle upwards. Ensure that you lift the point as much as possible before needling. Again, needle bilaterally, with evens technique.

Angle: 45-degree angle to the face.

See Figure 4.11.

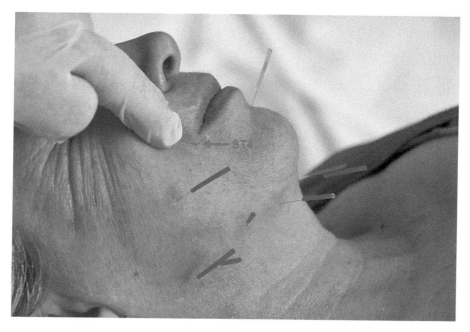

FIGURE 4.11 DEMONSTRATING NEEDLING AT ST4

LI20

Needle size: 25mm (length) × 0,16mm (thickness)/40 (gauge).

Technique: Needle bilaterally and using evens technique. This is the first point that we use to begin to lift and shape the cheek.

See Figure 4.12.

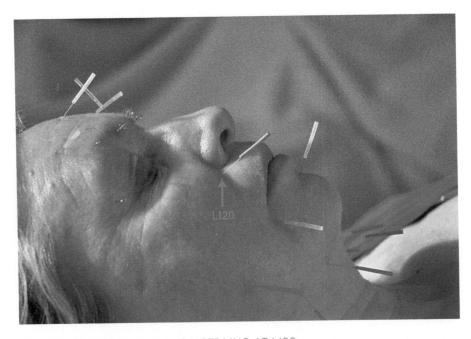

FIGURE 4.12 DEMONSTRATING NEEDLING AT LI20

ST3

Needle size: 25mm (length) × 0,16mm (thickness)/40 (gauge).

Technique: This is the second point used to shape the cheek area and it is needled perpendicularly and bilaterally, using evens technique.

See Figure 4.13.

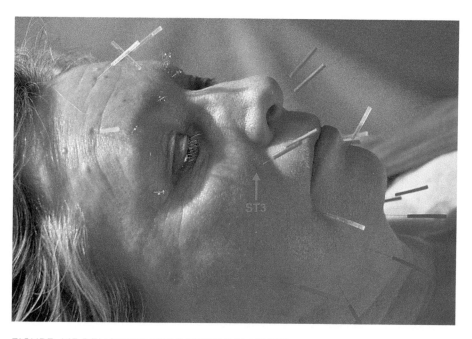

FIGURE 4.13 DEMONSTRATING NEEDLING AT ST3

SI18

Needle size: 25mm (length) × 0,16mm (thickness)/40 (gauge).

Technique: The third location forming the triangle of cheek-sculpting points. Needle bilaterally, using evens technique.

See Figure 4.14.

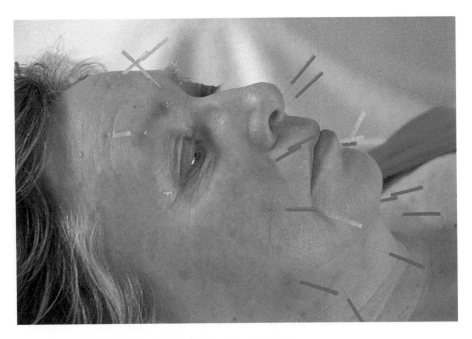

FIGURE 4.14 DEMONSTRATING NEEDLING AT SI18

ST2

Needle size: 15mm (length) × 0,20mm (thickness)/36 (gauge).

Technique: Evens and needled bilaterally.

See Figure 4.15.

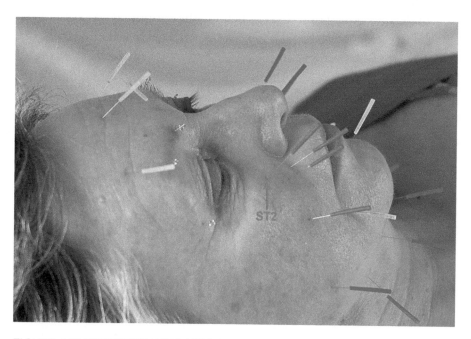

FIGURE 4.15 DEMONSTRATING NEEDLING AT ST2

4.3.9 NEEDLING THE CHIN

Ren 24

Needle size: 15mm (length) × 0,20mm (thickness)/36 (gauge).

Technique: Evens.

See Figure 4.16.

4.3.10 TREATING THE NECK

I generally use the first three points during every treatment that I perform. ST13 and GB21 are optional and are added to the protocol when the patient wants particular attention given to their neck area.

SI17

Needle size: 25mm (length) × 0,16mm (thickness)/40 (gauge).

Technique: This technique is very effective for tightening the neck muscles. When needling this point in a facial treatment, needle in the direction of (not under the skin) point TH17, behind the earlobe. If the patient has excess skin there, pinch the flesh together as you needle and implement this step with extreme caution. This is a vulnerable part of the neck and must be needled with great care. Aim to achieve a 'grabbing' sensation. When needled correctly, the muscles will be taut and there will be a significant improvement to the appearance of the neck area. Needle bilaterally with an evens technique.

Angle: 45 degrees.

See Figure 4.17.

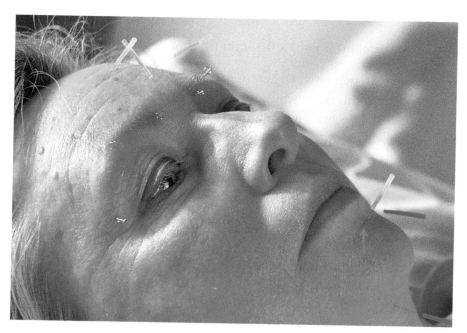

FIGURE 4.16 DEMONSTRATING NEEDLING AT REN 24

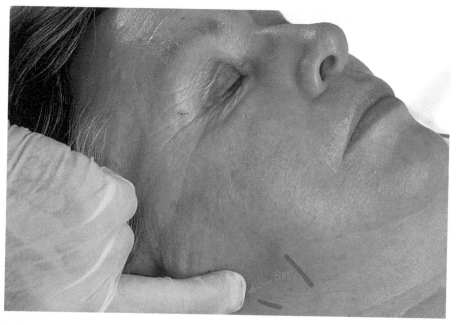

FIGURE 4.17 DEMONSTRATING NEEDLING AT SI17

Ren 23

Needle size: 25mm (length) × 0,16mm (thickness)/40 (gauge).

Technique: This point is listed here due to its location on the neck, although I tend to needle this point whilst working on the jaw points, as it is in the same area and it seems a natural progression. Ren 23 should be needled with an evens technique.

See Figure 4.18.

ST9

Needle size: 25mm (length) × 0,16mm (thickness)/40 (gauge).

Technique: Tonification and bilaterally.

See Figure 4.19.

ST13

Needle size: 25mm (length) × 0,16mm (thickness)/40 (gauge).

Technique: Tonification and bilaterally.

Note: Needle with extreme caution.

GB21

Needle size: 25mm (length) × 0,16mm (thickness)/40 (gauge).

Technique: Tonification and bilaterally.

Note: Contraindicated in pregnancy.

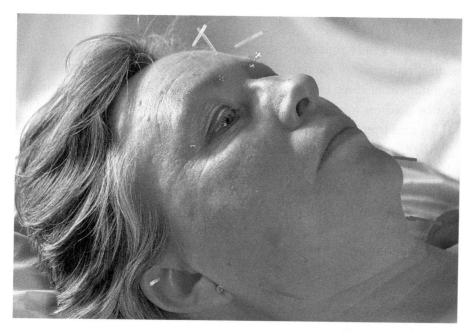

FIGURE 4.18 DEMONSTRATING NEEDLING AT REN 23

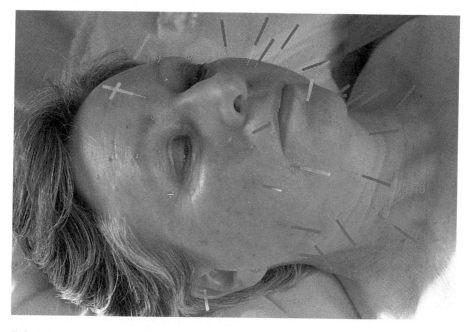

FIGURE 4.19 DEMONSTRATING NEEDLING AT ST9

4.3.11 TREATING WRINKLES

Treating lines and wrinkles on the face using Facial Enhancement Acupuncture is an effective part of the protocol and one that should give good results after a minimum of three treatments. The same intradermal needling technique can be used on forehead lines and also areas such as the nasal labial fold, which runs from the side of the nose to the corner of the mouth.

The latter, along with the 'number elevens' (lines between the eyes at the bridge of the nose), are two of the most commonly requested areas of the face that I am asked to treat. Known as glabellar frown lines, the 'number elevens' are formed by the movement of the underlying *procerus* and *corrugator supercilli* muscles. Sun exposure and genetics are a cause, along with too much frowning. This may sound odd, but many of us have jobs that involve staring at a computer screen all day and even the fine needling we perform as acupuncturists requires a lot of concentration. Of course, we all grow older and, as we do, the collagen and elastin production in our skin reduces.

Other areas that benefit from treatment can be the 'crow's feet' lines around the eyes, although I prefer to call them the starburst lines! And, of course, the lines that appear across the forehead can be especially deep on some patients, depending on their exposure to the sun and the elements.

From my experience, it is possible to make a difference to any of these areas using facial acupuncture, but obviously some parts of the face will respond better than others. If the line is particularly deep, it may take a lot more than three treatments to have any profound effect. Having said that, providing you and your patient are prepared to work on the area over a course of time, you will start to see some quite dramatic results.

Obviously, the ageing process plays a huge part in getting wrinkles, but why is this?

As we age, our facial bone structure starts to shrink; couple this with the loss of collagen and elasticity in the face, add in gravity and what we have as a result are wrinkles. Genetics are always going to be a factor in how we age, but there are many external factors that contribute to the speed at which this happens. A major cause of wrinkles that I often come across is, of course, sun damage. This was highlighted in a 2010 study, which examined the skin of participants who had been exposed to the sun for a large proportion of their life through a nearby window, due to their occupation or activities:

> Significant differences were observed in clinical scores for wrinkles, skin roughness assessed by fringe projection on the cheek, and skin heterogeneity assessed with spectrocolorimetry on the cheekbone. Other differences were observed for skin hydration, as well as skin laxity, which tended towards significance. (Mac-Mary *et al.* 2010, p.277)

The sun will affect people in varying ways depending on the amount of melanin that they have in their skin.

Smoking is a well-known major factor that causes wrinkles on the face, and it can be very evident on the top lip of those who have smoked for a number of years. It is, however, not solely the repetitive action of smoking that adds to the lines and wrinkles, but what the cigarette is doing to the body and the pollutants in tobacco smoke. An interesting study carried out in 2004 was the first to examine whether there was an earlier need for cosmetic surgery in smokers. A questionnaire was sent to 517 patients who had undergone blepharoplasy (upper-eyelid correction) due to valid dermatochalasis or 'baggy eyes': 'The smokers underwent surgery an average of 3.7 years earlier than the ex-smokers and 3.5 years earlier than the never-smokers' (Deliaert *et al.* 2012, p.853).

Ideally, if my patient has made the decision to stop smoking and would like me to help, I will work with them using traditional acupuncture before commencing with a course of facial acupuncture.

It is so often overlooked, but one of my top ten anti-ageing tips is simply to drink enough water. Loss of hydration can affect the skin in many ways, such as flakiness, tightness and dryness. Dry skin is particularly more prone to fine lines and wrinkles.

Drinking sufficient water is also important for removal of waste from the body. If the volume of fluid is decreased, then the body finds it much more difficult to remove toxins. This can result in the body attempting to expel them through the skin, which can in turn exacerbate conditions such as eczema and acne. I always recommend that my patients maintain an adequate intake of water throughout the day.

So, how much is adequate? The recommended daily amount of water is eight glasses a day, but that has been subject to a lot of criticism. As with everything, we are all unique, and different people may require varying levels of water depending on the local climate, activity, type of job, age, sex, weight, food intake and alcohol and so on.

I am able to use the information derived from the initial consultation to establish whether a couple more glasses a day may benefit my patient's health and their skin. One suggestion could be that your patient drinks enough to ensure that their urine is mostly clear.

Personally, I use a distiller in my clinic, as I believe this is preferable to tap water. So, the quality of water is important to think about too.

As acupuncturists, looking at our patient's diet and lifestyle will already be integral and these skills can be incorporated into your cosmetic treatments, ensuring we are always working from the inside out.

So, we have looked at the potential causes and how we can help to prevent deep lines and wrinkles forming. However, we will now concentrate on the method for needling the lines and wrinkles that our patients are looking for us to treat.

Intradermal Needling
Needles: 6mm intradermal.

Technique: We will be using tweezers to insert these needles, as we did for the three eyebrow points. Remove the intradermal needle from its individual packaging with the tweezers. You will need to practise holding the intradermals with the tweezers. The first time you use them it will feel a little strange, but once you have carried out a few treatments they will become second nature.

When the appropriate number of intradermals have been inserted into the target line, they need to be left in position for at least 20 minutes. During this time a redness or erythema will appear around the needled area. This shows us that the treatment is working.

When you remove the intradermals with your tweezers, it is always worth having a cotton bud on standby to help extract the needle. Sometimes, you will find that the intradermals tend to grab the skin and you will need to put a little pressure at the base of the needle to help with its removal. By doing this you will also help to prevent bruising.

After treating any areas with intradermal needles, you will usually see some improvement after a minimum of three treatments. A course of ten treatments is recommended for optimum results, followed by maintenance treatments every few months. The latter will help to prolong the effects of the initial treatments and ensure the fine lines and wrinkles remain diminished.

NUMBER ELEVENS

Begin with the lines in between the eyebrows at the bridge of the nose. Look at one of the lines that you want to needle; you will need to open the line up by using two fingers of the opposite hand that you are needling with. We want to insert the needle into the base of the line; if you visualise the line or wrinkle as a narrow canyon, the needle needs to go right into the bottom of the canyon. Insert the intradermal needles at a 45-degree angle to the skin; the needles should be spaced at about 2mm intervals. The direction of the needle is not overly important, but on these 'number elevens' I still try to work in an upward direction. If we are looking at a line approximately 2.5cm in length, we should be trying to insert at least ten intradermals. The needles should be inserted to a depth that is comfortable to the patient. This need not be the full depth of the needle shaft; however, try to maintain the 45-degree angle as you needle. See Figure 4.20.

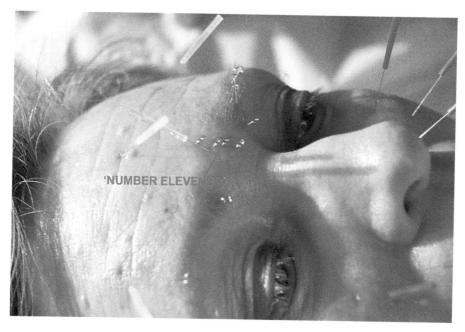

FIGURE 4.20 DEMONSTRATING INTRADERMAL NEEDLING AT THE 'NUMBER ELEVENS'

FOREHEAD

Again, you will need to insert your needles at a spacing of 2mm and work across the line from one end to the other. This is one of the rare occasions when we are not needling in an upward direction. When needling the forehead lines, we are attempting to insert as much of the intradermal needle shaft into the skin and along the line as possible. Aim to maintain a 45-degree angle from the forehead as you needle. Be patient. The more intradermals you can insert into the line, the better the overall outcome. See Figures 4.21 and 4.22.

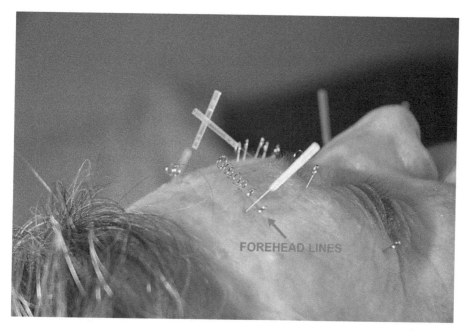

FIGURE 4.21 A CLOSE-UP OF INTRADERMAL
NEEDLING IN A FOREHEAD LINE

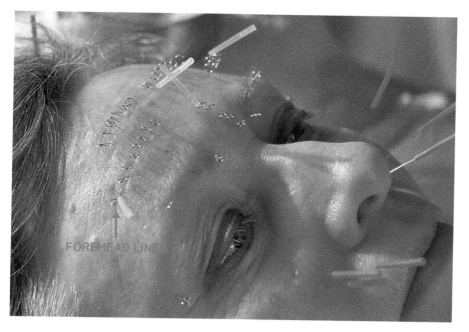

FIGURE 4.22 DEMONSTRATING INTRADERMAL
NEEDLING IN THE FOREHEAD LINES

NASAL LABIAL FOLD

The nasal labial fold between the corner of the mouth and the side of the nose can be treated in exactly the same way. Again, make sure that the line is opened up, so that you can needle directly into the base of it. Practise opening the line with the forefinger and thumb of one hand as you needle with the other. This makes the insertion of the intradermals a lot easier than when the skin is loose. Spacing of the intradermal needles should be approximately 2mm apart and again I would needle in an upward direction. See Figures 4.23 and 4.24.

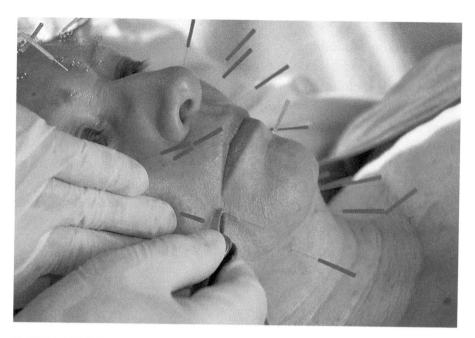

FIGURE 4.23 DEMONSTRATING THE INTRADERMAL NEEDLING
TECHNIQUE AT THE BASE OF THE NASAL LABIAL FOLD

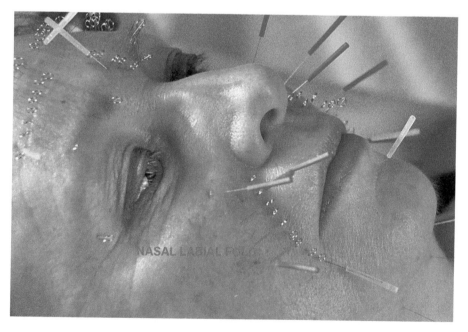

FIGURE 4.24 DEMONSTRATING INTRADERMAL NEEDLING ALONG
THE NASAL LABIAL FOLD

CROW'S FEET

When working around the eyes, we need to take extra care as this area can be very sensitive and we do not want to needle too close to the eye. From experience, if there is any chance of bruising, this is the most likely area where it will happen. If you do bruise the patient, do not panic. Have some arnica cream on hand and apply this to the skin as soon as the bruise appears.

Using your usual technique of opening up the line with one hand, insert the intradermal needle gently into the line around the eye. As always, try to maintain a 45-degree angle from the skin and insert the needles towards the eye. See Figure 4.25.

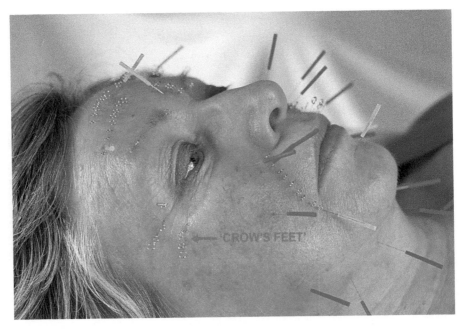

FIGURE 4.25 DEMONSTRATING INTRADERMAL NEEDLING ON THE 'CROW'S FEET'

TOP LIP

This is another area that is very popular for treatment. Patients very often complain about the lines that appear here which, as we discussed earlier, are often, but not always, caused by smoking. Using the intradermal needles is a very effective way of addressing these lines, but this area can be particularly sensitive. The anaesthetic points that we have needled should be sufficient but, if a lot of work is required in this area, it may be appropriate to apply the anaesthetic cream before you commence the protocol to assist with this.

After needling the top lip area, you can then take a little more time to address any other fine lines and wrinkles, such as those on the chin and across the bridge of the nose. See Figure 4.26.

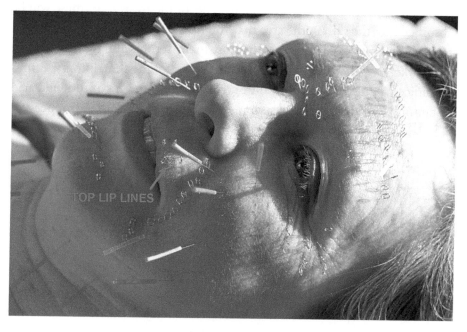

FIGURE 4.26 DEMONSTRATING INTRADERMAL NEEDLING ALONG THE TOP LIP, CHIN AND THE BRIDGE OF THE NOSE

HOW IT WORKS

The action of using the intradermal needles is two-fold. First, by inserting the needle, we are creating a very small injury to the skin. The body then produces collagen that repairs this injury and, due to the location of the needle insertion, this will start to fill out the line. Second, we have created a number of small perforations in the skin along the line that we are treating; these perforations will remain open for a short while, which will give us the opportunity to apply skin rejuvenating serums and moisturisers that will be absorbed into the upper layers of the dermis.

4.3.12 APPLYING SERUMS AND CREAMS

Remove all of the needles inserted from Steps 4.3.2–4.3.11 in reverse to the order they were inserted. Use the tweezers to remove the intradermal needles and gently press down on the skin with a cotton bud as you remove each one, to prevent bruising. Retain the needles in the hands, arms, feet and legs; these will be removed at the end of the treatment (see Section 4.5).

We now have a small window of time to apply any serums or moisturisers to the area in order to maximise the benefits of the treatment; these will be absorbed into the skin in the area that you have needled and aid in the skin's rejuvenation process. Of course, there are many serums and moisturisers on the market that all profess to improve the quality of the skin, but my serums of choice would either be a hyaluronic acid serum, with pantothenic acid (vitamin B5) and/or a retinol serum. These are applied with a dropper and are concentrated, so they need to be used sparingly and gently massaged into the face following treatment. Allow the serums to sink into the skin, before moving on to the next step.

Hyaluronic Acid

This sounds like the last thing you would want to administer to a patient's face, but it is actually extremely gentle and is 'naturally present in the skin as part of the extracellular matrix and as a component of collagen'. John and Price go on to say that it also 'acts as a ground substance of the dermis, and is also a component of joint fluid, vitreous of eye, disc nucleus, and the umbilical cord' (John and Price 2009, p.226).

One of the most significant properties of hyaluronic acid is 'its capacity to bind huge amounts of water (1000-fold of its own weight)' (Jiang, Liang and Noble 2007, p.437). As this is a natural molecule, which decreases as we age, it is one of the reasons that skin becomes dry and joints stiffen. Applying this to the face after needling greatly improves absorption and allows the hyaluronic acid to penetrate the dermis more deeply. Due to its massive hydrating capacity, this, in turn, provides additional moisture which works to plump and smooth out the wrinkles.

Pantothenic Acid

This is also known as vitamin B5 and is often found alongside hyaluronic acid in readily available serums for external use. This water-soluble vitamin is one of the three components of *Coenzyme A* occurring naturally in the body.

Dr Lit-Hung Leung investigated vitamin B5 for the treatment of acne vulgaris. Participants were asked to take an extremely high dose daily and also apply a topical solution which contained pantothenic acid. Within only two to three days, there was a visible reduction in facial sebum secretion and the condition was found to be under control after eight weeks. The other facial benefit was the shrinking pores:

> The pore size becomes noticeably smaller within 1–2 weeks, very often much sooner. Like sebum excretion, the pores will continue to shrink until the skin becomes much finer, giving the patient a much more beautiful skin. (Leung 1997, p.106)

This study demonstrates the beneficial effects of pantothenic acid for acne sufferers and, although we are only applying it topically, vitamin B5 will still have a beneficial effect on the patient's skin.

We discussed in Section 4.3.11 how we are making very tiny injuries when we needle the skin, which will encourage collagen induction to plump the wrinkles. Pantothenic acid is widely known for its wound-healing properties as it 'aids in the production of the lipoproteins of the skin, hastening its healing time' (Sharma *et al.* 2011, p.1520). This is why

I choose to apply this vitamin as part of a serum that contains hyaluronic acid. After all of the intradermal needling we have carried out, this acts as a natural hydrating and healing part of the treatment.

Retinol

Also known as vitamin A, retinol has some key functions in the body relating to embryology and vision, through to immunity. Aside from these important roles, it is well known as an active ingredient in skin creams and serums. A 2007 randomised, double-blind, vehicle-controlled study evaluated the effectiveness of topical retinol in improving naturally aged skin: 'Topical retinol improves fine wrinkles associated with natural aging. Significant induction of glycosaminoglycan, which is known to retain substantial water, and increased collagen production are most likely responsible for wrinkle effacement' (Kafi *et al.* 2007, p.606).

A biologically active cosmeceutical such as all-trans-retinol (containing 0.3% retinol) is recommended and needs to be applied sparingly. While vitamin A is important to the body, it can be toxic in high doses and can also have a drying effect, so, if using retinol, you may want to include hyaluronic acid serum to lock in the moisture.

Note: Facial Enhancement Acupuncture is contraindicated for patients actively trying for a baby, pregnant or breast-feeding (see Section 4.1 for contraindications) and retinol should not be applied in any of these cases. Vitamin A is also not recommended for patients undergoing skin peeling procedures or taking medication prescribed for acne.

4.4 FACIAL ENHANCEMENT ACUPRESSURE MASSAGE

Many students on my courses have asked me whether the massage part of my treatment protocol is that important. Of course, it is entirely up to you as a practitioner as to which elements you choose to include in your treatments. However, my advice would be to include a massage of one type or another that will provide a conclusion to the treatment. I cannot profess to be a qualified masseur, but it has been worth my time and effort to investigate ways of improving this aspect of the treatment. If you spend some time investigating what works for you, then I believe it will be time well spent.

When you start to look into facial massage as a subject in its own right, you will find that there are many books written on the topic and many practitioners specialising in this form of treatment. Working with the facial muscles of a patient using massage has, for a long time, been recognised as a way of delaying the ageing process and improving the patient's facial appearance. If you then consider that with acupuncture we are working with those same muscle groups, but to a far greater depth than just massage, then it is hardly surprising that we should be getting such good results.

My patients really enjoy their facial massage and it also provides an opportunity for me to analyse their face and plan what I would like to work on at their next treatment session. I will go through a few of the massage techniques that I use and then leave it up to you to do your own investigation. What I am about to describe here should be enough to get you started.

Before we start on the facial massage, we need to make sure our patient is happy and relaxed. This should be a pleasurable experience for them and not just a rushed procedure at the end of a treatment protocol. Using acupressure points during the massage also gives the added benefit of helping to lift the face and benefit the work that we have already achieved with the needles.

It is very important to use a good-quality base cream when you are massaging the face. Your fingers need to be able to move freely across the skin and not drag at any point. Do not be afraid to use some pressure on the face. From experience, patients prefer some gentle pressure during a massage, rather than a delicate tickling-type sensation. I use a natural anti-inflammatory cream with vitamin E for the facial massage. This can be applied once any serums you have chosen to use have had a little time to sink into the skin. The anti-inflammatory helps to promote skin healing following needling and the vitamin E nourishes the skin. An alternative might be to use a natural collagen-based cream to further boost the collagen-induction aspects of the treatment. Alternatively, you may already prepare your own aromatherapy creams and would prefer to work with these.

I have broken my signature Facial Enhance massage down into some very easy steps. Feel free to mix them up and add in anything of your own, but it is always important to have a basic structure to what you are trying to achieve. I can honestly say that if you take your time with this part of the treatment protocol, it will cement the good work that you have done with the needles and you will end up with some remarkable results.

4.4.1 MASSAGE STAGE 1

Begin your facial massage by gently placing both thumbs on a point approximately 1.5 cun above Yin Tang. Apply a gentle rocking motion in this position, along with upward pressure. Then, after a few seconds, gently slide both thumbs outwards towards the edges of the forehead. As you do this, apply a gentle amount of pressure to smooth the brow lines and any forehead lines or creases. See Figures 4.27 and 4.28.

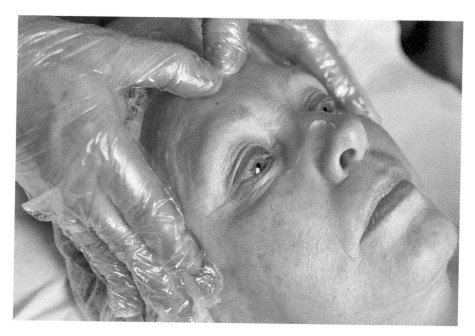

FIGURE 4.27 PLACING THUMBS ABOVE YIN TANG
TO BEGIN THE FACIAL MASSAGE

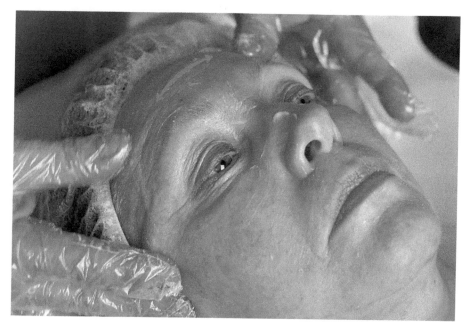

FIGURE 4.28 SLIDING BOTH THUMBS ACROSS THE FOREHEAD

Once you have massaged the forehead a few times using this technique, let your thumbs come to rest on your patient's temple area, just above the end of the eyebrow. Now, applying a gentle pressure and using a circular motion, massage this area for a few seconds. See Figure 4.29.

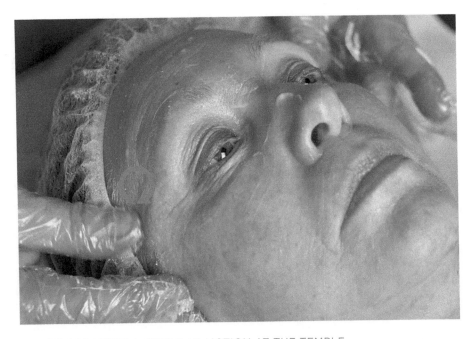

FIGURE 4.29 USING A CIRCULAR MOTION AT THE TEMPLE

4.4.2 MASSAGE STAGE 2

Using the second finger of your right hand, apply pressure to the middle of your patient's left eyebrow at the point Yuyao. Gently slide your finger towards the top of the patient's forehead, lifting the eyebrow as you do so. As your finger reaches the top of the forehead, do exactly the same with the middle finger of your other hand. Continue with this relatively quick motion, one after another for a few seconds. By doing this you will stimulate the muscles in the forehead that raise the eyebrows. Move to the right side and repeat. This same technique is very effective when used on the area above Yin Tang, in between the eyebrows. Use a gentle pressure to smooth this area towards the hairline. See Figure 4.30.

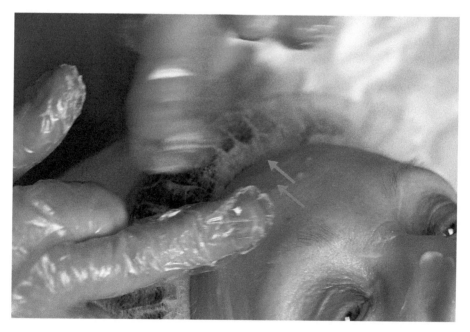

FIGURE 4.30 USING THE MIDDLE FINGERS TO MASSAGE THE FOREHEAD WITH CONTINUOUS STROKES

4.4.3 MASSAGE STAGE 3

Using the thumbs of both hands, position the pads of the thumbs directly on acupuncture point LI20. Apply some gentle pressure on this point for at least ten seconds and then softly smooth the nasal labial fold from top to bottom using the thumb. See Figures 4.31 and 4.32.

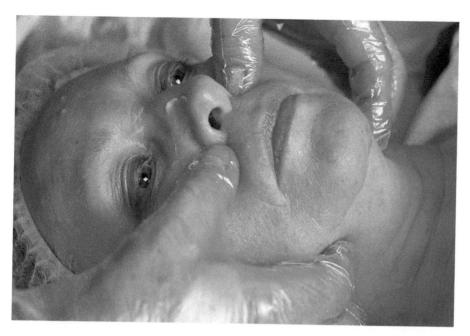

FIGURE 4.31 BEGIN BY PLACING YOUR THUMBS AT LI20

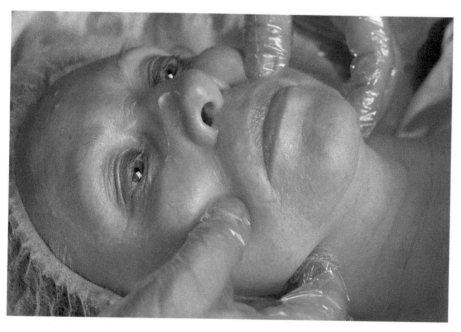

FIGURE 4.32 SWEEP DOWN THE NASAL LABIAL FOLD

4.4.4 MASSAGE STAGE 4

While we are at the corner of the mouth, following Stage 3, apply upward pressure to pressure point ST4 for approximately ten seconds. See Figure 4.33.

Using a similar amount of pressure as used on ST4, at this stage we need to apply downward pressure on points ST3 and SI18. Use the tip of the fingers and apply the pressure for approximately ten seconds; these points are great for shaping the cheekbone area.

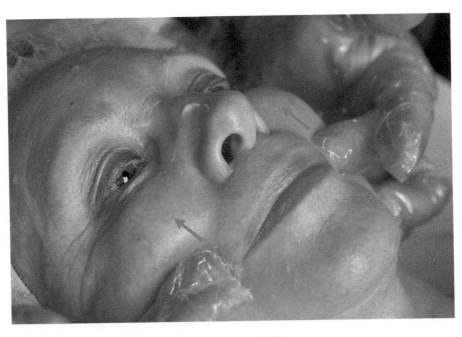

FIGURE 4.33 APPLYING PRESSURE TO POINT ST4

4.4.5 MASSAGE STAGE 5

We now turn our attention to the area just below the bottom lip. We are going to be stimulating the pressure point Ren 24. Using both thumbs and a gentle lifting and stroking action, massage this point by alternating from one thumb to the other for a few seconds. See Figure 4.34.

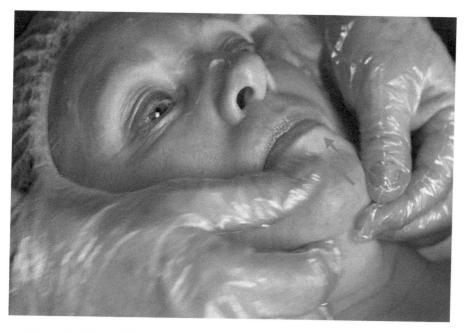

FIGURE 4.34 CONTINUOUSLY STROKING THE CHIN IN AN UPWARDS DIRECTION USING EACH THUMB

Move your hands down to your patient's neck and position both thumbs either side of pressure point ST9. Now, with long gentle sweeping strokes, massage the patient's neck from ST9 up to just below the ears. See Figures 4.35, 4.36 and 4.37.

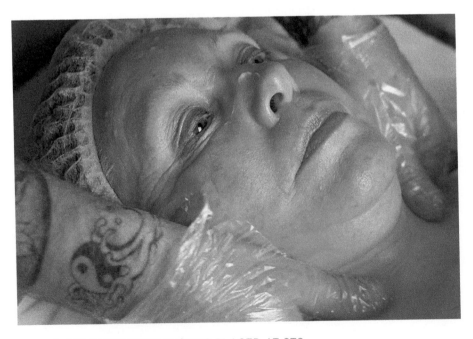

FIGURE 4.35 BEGIN WITH THUMBS PLACED AT ST9

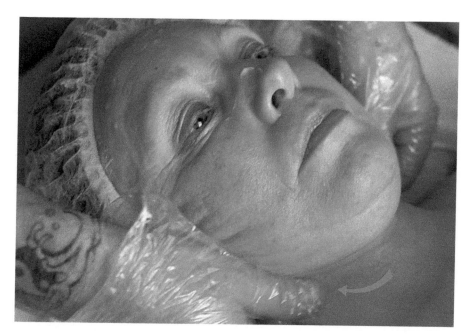

FIGURE 4.36 GENTLY SWEEPING THE THUMBS UP THE NECK

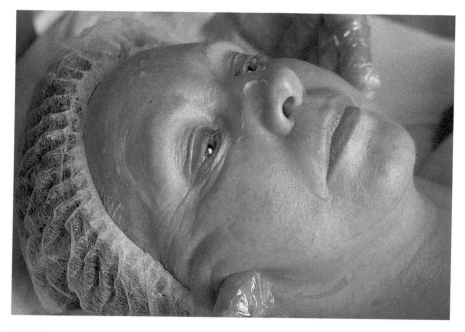

FIGURE 4.37 FINISHING THE STROKE FROM ST9 BENEATH THE EARS

4.4.6 MASSAGE STAGE 6

Using the thumbs, and also the fleshy part at the base of the thumbs, apply pressure to your patient's face directly below the eyes at ST2 and then move to the side of the ears. Carefully pull back on the patient's cheek towards the ears and hold the tension for ten seconds. Repeat this three times on both sides. See Figure 4.38.

To bring the facial massage to an end, use both hands to apply long upward sweeping strokes to your patient's neck. Keep contact with your patient at all times as this makes them feel secure and the massage is more relaxing. See Figures 4.39 and 4.40.

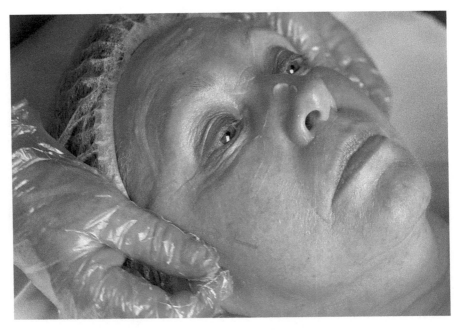

FIGURE 4.38 HOLDING THE TENSION ON THE CHEEKS UP TOWARDS THE EARS

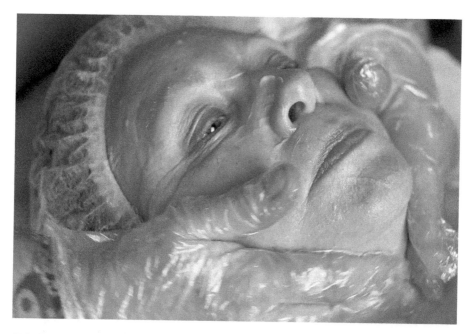

FIGURE 4.39 PLACING BOTH HANDS, WITH FINGERS TOUCHING AT THE CENTRE OF THE NECK

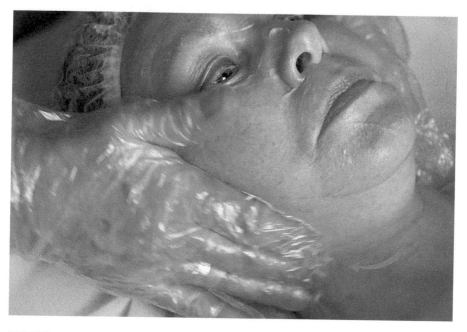

FIGURE 4.40 SWEEPING UPWARD STROKES ON THE NECK AREA

Finally, massage in a good-quality moisturiser. Again, the choice of moisturiser is entirely up to you and warrants some research. However, I would recommend sourcing a product that is perfume- and paraben-free. You may be treating some patients with sensitive skin and a gentle, yet potent, high-quality cosmeticeutical will be less likely to cause a reaction. Your treatment results will also be enhanced by using a cream with premium ingredients. I use a natural, hydrating, pro-collagen moisturiser, at this stage, which contains retinyl palmitate (vitamin A derivative). I find this the perfect finish for my treatment as it helps to lock in moisture and promote collagen synthesis.

4.5 FINISHING THE TREATMENT

The full Facial Enhancement Acupuncture protocol is now complete and you can set about removing the final needles that you inserted in Steps 4.3.2 and 4.3.3.

Leave your patient to relax for a few minutes, as they have received a somewhat intensive treatment. There has been a lot of facial work carried out and their skin should look vibrant, but they will be able to appreciate the effects more fully within a few hours once their face has completely settled down.

Encourage your patient to refrain from touching their face, where possible, immediately following their treatment, to ensure the skin remains clean after the needling.

CHAPTER 5

ADVANCED FACIAL ENHANCEMENT TECHNIQUES

5.1 JADE GUA SHA
5.1.1 ABOUT GUA SHA

Gua Sha is an East Asian treatment which generally uses quite a vigorous rubbing/scraping technique. It is mainly used in China on the patient's back, for detoxification purposes or for various sprains and injuries throughout the body. Gua means 'to scrape or scratch' and Sha is the resulting redness or rash (Nielsen 1995, p.43).

We are going to be using a Chinese jade Gua Sha stone to massage our patient's face and to help our serums and creams penetrate the skin more deeply. The first thing to mention is that, to be accurate, my technique is not considered a true Gua Sha technique, in the sense of those practised for thousands of years. The original Gua Sha method uses much more intense stimulation along the acupuncture meridians and clears areas of stagnation on a patient's body. This treatment is fairly strong and creates the redness on the patient's skin that we have described. Obviously, we do not want to use this type of technique on the face, which would be too sensitive for authentic Gua Sha. The facial version that we use requires extreme care, as the skin on the face is far more delicate. Used in this way, it is a lovely, relaxing part of the treatment that can again be used across the cheeks, around the eyes, on the forehead, the nasal labial fold and the fine lines around the mouth.

When working on the face, I use a jade Gua Sha stone, mainly because of its cooling properties. My stone of choice is a beautiful, smooth piece of jade that is carved in such a way that it fits into the various angles of the face. This means that I can use the stone to massage the areas that I might struggle to get to using hands alone. However, Gua Sha is often practised with regular day-to-day objects such as spoons or coins. The best way to use the stone is to combine it with a good-quality cream that nourishes the skin and enables smooth movement of the tool. The important thing to remember when using Gua Sha on the face is to make sure the pressure that you apply is enough to help the serums and creams penetrate the skin, but not too heavy that it is an uncomfortable experience for the patient.

5.1.2 THE GUA SHA FACIAL MASSAGE

If you opt to include Gua Sha in your treatment, I would recommend adding it in before the facial massage outlined in Section 4.4. First, apply a liberal amount of your serum of choice (for instance, hyaluronic acid) to the areas of the face that you intend to massage. Allow this to sink in and then apply some massage cream to the same areas; this cream is what will allow the Gua Sha stone to move freely over the face (see Section 4.4 for further information about massage cream).

Use the large smooth edge of the stone in long sweeping strokes to massage from the neck right up to just below the ears. See Figure 5.1.

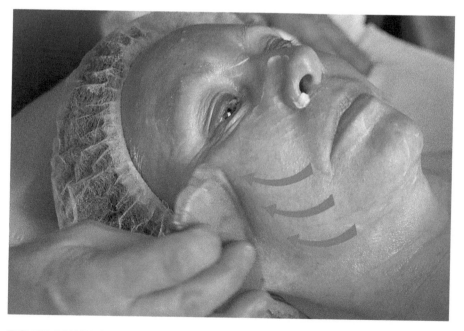

FIGURE 5.1 USING GENTLE PRESSURE TO SWEEP THE JADE GUA SHA STONE FROM THE NECK TO THE EAR

Aside from this, I do not sweep the stone in any particular direction. For instance, when I concentrate the tool on the nasal labial fold, I use it within the fold itself, beginning with a gentle rocking motion and building to more circular sweeping strokes along the line. See Figure 5.2.

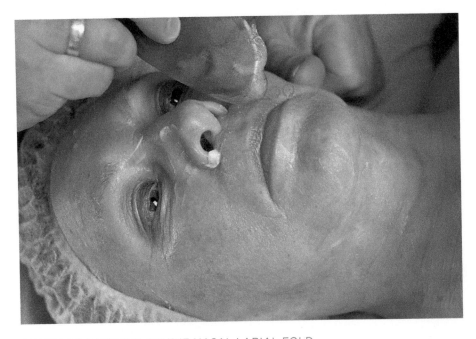

FIGURE 5.2 WORKING ON THE NASAL LABIAL FOLD

As I work along each line, I am using the Gua Sha stone almost like an eraser, but with a gentle circular motion to work the cream into the lines and wrinkles. See Figure 5.3.

I have found that the best results with this technique can often be found on the 'crow's feet' around the eyes. There are, however, no set rules or actions to using facial Gua Sha. As a practitioner, you need to practise your skills to achieve a pleasurable massage for your patient. My only comment is always to concentrate on massaging in an upward direction as, at all stages, we are attempting to lift the patient's face. What you are trying to do is encourage the muscles under the skin to tighten and, in turn, raise the face and reduce the lines. Also, you are aiming to get the energy moving in the face, as this has benefits for the circulation. A 2007 study found that Gua Sha 'increases microcirculation local to a treated area' (Nielsen *et al.* 2007, p.456). You will find that, with only very mild rubbing, the skin may redden. That is the Sha appearing and this will settle down within a couple of minutes. As long as you are using only a light pressure, the skin will respond well and your patient will feel very relaxed.

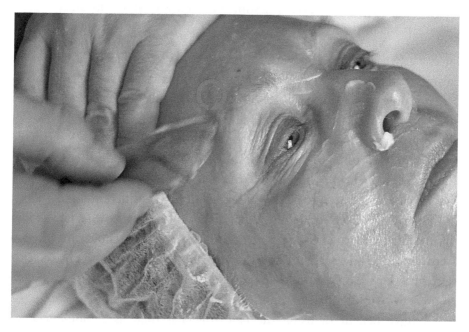

FIGURE 5.3 MASSAGING THE FOREHEAD LINES WITH THE TIP OF THE GUA SHA STONE

To keep my jade Gua Sha tool scrupulously clean between patients, I use a disinfecting jar. These are commonly found at hairdressing salons and are used to disinfect scissors, combs and so on. I keep this jar in my clinic room, so that my patients can see that the jade rollers, tweezers and Gua Sha stone, which we are using throughout their treatment, are all perfectly clean.

Gua Sha is an add-on to the Jade Roller Facial Enhancement Massage treatment and I usually dedicate around 5–10 minutes to this technique. Many of my patients have been very impressed by the treatment as it is soothing, yet works to tighten the whole face. Combining Gua Sha with a Facial Enhancement Acupuncture treatment can provide even more evident results.

5.2 JADE ROLLERS
5.2.1 ABOUT JADE ROLLERS

> Jade, which the Chinese have exalted for nearly 4000 years as
> their 'Jewel of Heaven,' is still, even in the West, the mystery
> stone of the ages. (Zara 2001, p.9)

It was my privilege to discover these rollers a few years ago and I have been using them in my cosmetic acupuncture treatments ever since. Jade rollers are not only lovely things to use but they are also very pleasing to the eye; they have a luxurious feel to them and are steeped in hundreds of years of history: 'For many centuries before or after Confucius (551–479 BC), jade was considered to be of supernatural origin, and to contain the essence of life, virtue and eternity' (Lyons 1978, p.6).

Usually, a set of jade rollers will comprise two different-sized rollers, although I have seen some rollers that are double-ended, with a large roller at one end and a smaller one at the other. My rollers of choice are the two separate rollers. The larger one is for use on the forehead and cheeks; it is also ideal for use on the neck. The second roller, which is quite a bit smaller, is great for working on the top lip and around the nose.

A huge benefit of using the jade rollers is that, as a 'side-effect' of treatment, many of my patients find that sinus problems they have been suffering from are diminished. Not only that, but because we are spending time rolling the face and neck, this aids lymphatic drainage, resulting in the body expelling a build-up of toxins: 'The lymphatic vascular system is essential for lipid absorption, fluid homeostasis, and immune surveillance' (Wang and Oliver 2010, p.2115). So, by rolling these lymph vessels and encouraging healthy flow, it can have a positive effect on overall health. This is one of the reasons that the Jade Roller Facial Enhancement Massage is so effective at reducing puffiness and oedema.

We have often heard of splashing cold water on our faces to close the pores, and the cooling jade is an ideal tool for achieving a similar effect following the treatment. As a result, I recommend adding the jade roller massage at the end of Section 4.4 (the Facial Enhancement Acupressure Massage) and before you moisturise the face.

5.2.2 STEP-BY-STEP JADE ROLLER FACIAL MASSAGE

I always begin with the large roller and, gently, with a little pressure, roll from the ear to the mouth and back again for approximately ten strokes on both sides of the face. See Figure 5.4.

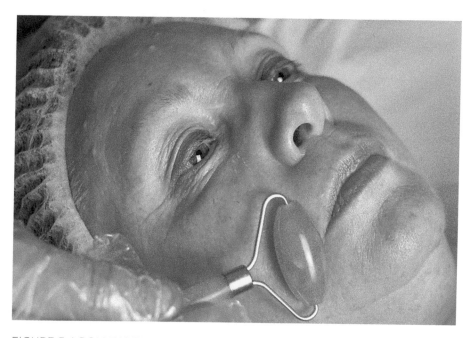

FIGURE 5.4 ROLLING THE JADE ROLLER FROM THE EAR TO THE MOUTH

Move the roller up the face and repeat the same technique, ensuring you roll right on to the nasal labial fold. See Figure 5.5.

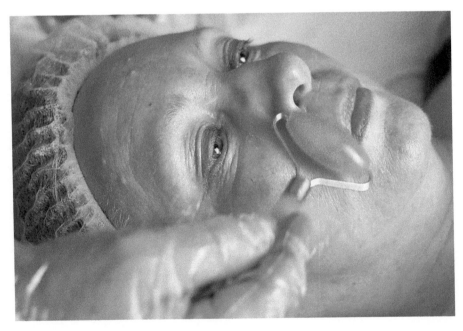

FIGURE 5.5 MOVING THE JADE ROLLER ACROSS TO FOCUS ON THE NASAL LABIAL FOLD

Next, begin to work on the neck, rolling from the lowest part of the neck, over the jaw and up to the ear in one long stroke. Always roll using upward strokes to lift this area and repeat on both sides. See Figure 5.6.

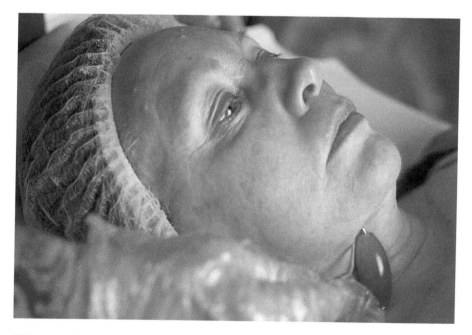

FIGURE 5.6 USING THE LARGE JADE ROLLER TO MASSAGE THE NECK

Then move to the eye area and carefully roll up and down by the side of the eye over the 'crow's feet' approximately ten times. Turning the roller 90 degrees, roll in the opposite direction. See Figures 5.7 and 5.8.

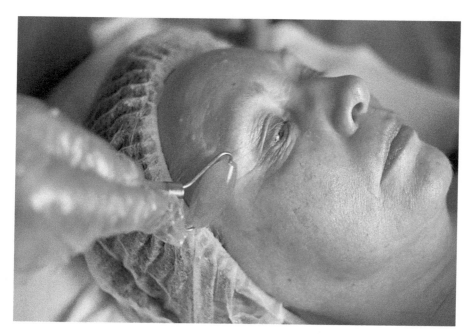

FIGURE 5.7 ROLLING THE LARGE JADE ROLLER
UP AND DOWN THE SIDE OF THE EYE

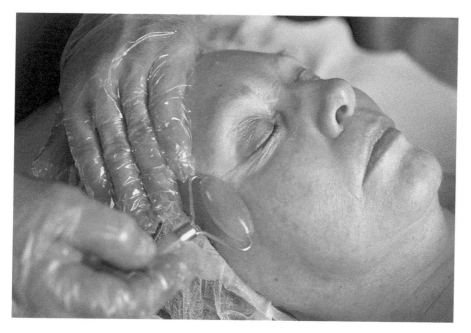

FIGURE 5.8 TURNING THE LARGE JADE ROLLER
90 DEGREES TO ROLL UP TO THE EYE

Finally, use the large roller to sweep across the front of the face, repeating the same method as before on both sides. See Figure 5.9.

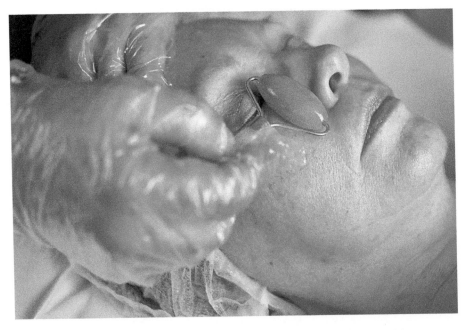

FIGURE 5.9 SWEEPING THE LARGE JADE ROLLER ACROSS THE FACE

Switching to the smaller roller enables you to work more thoroughly on the nasal labial fold. Roll back and forth across the line approximately 10–15 times on both sides. See Figure 5.10.

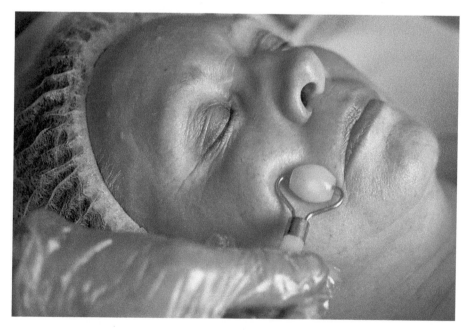

FIGURE 5.10 USING THE SMALL JADE ROLLER
TO ROLL ACROSS THE NASAL LABIAL FOLD

At this stage, you can roll across the chin approximately ten times, where you needled at Ren 24. See Figure 5.11.

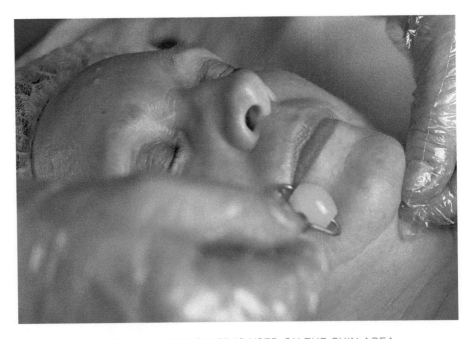

FIGURE 5.11 THE SMALL JADE ROLLER IS USED ON THE CHIN AREA

The smaller roller also enables you to get into the top lip area, where you can push the creams into the lines that form around the mouth. Roll back and forth across each side of the area for approximately ten strokes. See Figure 5.12.

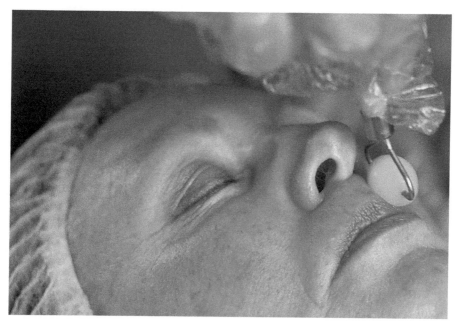

FIGURE 5.12 TARGETING THE TOP LIP AREA WITH THE SMALL JADE ROLLER

Next, move on to the eye area. We have already covered this section using the larger roller which massages this area as a whole, but we can really target the fine lines around the eye by using the small roller to gently traverse the 'crow's feet'. See Figure 5.13.

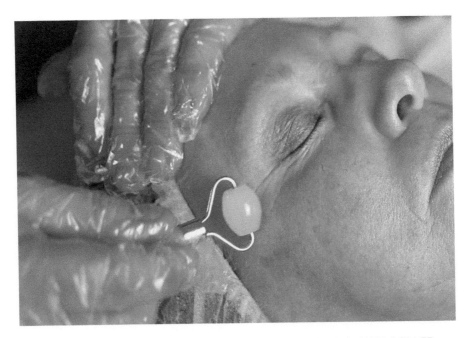

FIGURE 5.13 ROLLING THE 'CROW'S FEET' WITH THE SMALL JADE ROLLER

Finally, tend to the 'number elevens' and forehead lines by rolling up and down the area. Concentrate on the centre to begin with and continue the technique outwards across the forehead on either side, making sure to cover the whole expanse of the forehead from eyebrow to hairline. See Figure 5.14.

This completes the Jade Roller Massage and your patient should feel very relaxed following this stage of the treatment. Remember, if you have added this step into your treatment plan, this is the time to finalise the massage by applying moisturiser.

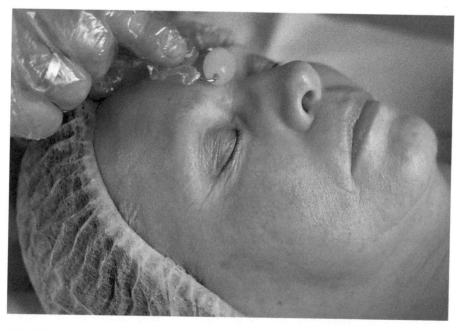

FIGURE 5.14 USING THE SMALL JADE ROLLER TO SMOOTH THE 'NUMBER ELEVENS'

5.3 DERMAL ROLLERS
5.3.1 ABOUT DERMAL ROLLERS

Micro Needle Therapy (MNT) or Dermal Rolling (also known as dermarolling, derma-rolling, skin needling and collagen induction therapy) is based on some of the same principles as facial acupuncture. This puts acupuncturists in the perfect place to consider offering this treatment in their practice.

The dermal roller is a plastic-handled tool with a rotating head that is covered in up to 200 micro needles. The top-quality rollers use titanium needles and the needle length for the rollers can vary from a fraction of a millimetre up to 3mm in length. My needle length of choice for facial treatments is a 1.5mm dermal roller. These rollers are sterile and disposable, intended for one-time use on your patient. Alternatively, you can opt to use a dermal pen, which is the latest development in this treatment sector. This is a tool that can be fitted with sterile, disposable needle heads. The electronic device can then be used to glide gently across the skin, whilst the vibrational movement vertically pierces the skin with the tiny micro needles.

Micro Needle Therapy should be looked at as an add-on treatment to your Facial Enhancement Acupuncture and, as such, full training in the use of dermal rollers should be attained before performing this treatment in your clinic. Therefore, this section will simply aim to provide information about this area of skin needling and how it can benefit your patients.

5.3.2 HOW SKIN NEEDLING WORKS

We have all injured ourselves in one way or another in the past and probably noticed how the wound or injury heals very quickly, usually leaving stronger tissue than before. This is the body's own healing mechanism, creating new collagen to repair itself. Just like in the intradermal needling technique, this intricate process is the basis behind MNT; we are creating the smallest of injuries to the face and letting our body do what it does best and heal the wounds. The only difference with the dermal roller or dermal pen and an acupuncture needle is that by the time we have completed an MNT treatment we have created over 2000 miniscule injuries that instantly begin to repair and rejuvenate. This repair and renew process is what makes MNT such an exciting development in natural cosmetic treatments.

Combine the effect of the small injuries to the face with the ability to introduce high-quality moisturisers and serums to the lower layer of the dermis of the skin and you have an all-round facial treatment that will provide impressive results. Due to the increased collagen production, the effects will continue to improve in the weeks and months after the treatment.

Many people have asked me to provide comparisons with MNT and other facial procedures. MNT is considered to be a 'nonablative' treatment that provides the same results as ablative treatments such as microdermabrasion and chemical peels. Benefits include rejuvenating ageing skin and diminishing the appearance of common skin conditions such as indented scars, large pores and/or uneven skin tone, but the method involved is different: 'As opposed to ablative laser treatments, the epidermis remains intact and is not damaged' (Aust *et al.* 2008, p.1421). The aim of this type of treatment is to induce new collagen production without the need to remove this outer layer of skin.

The topmost layer of the epidermis is known as the *stratum corneum*. It was viewed for many years as a dead layer of skin, but its intrinsic role as a barrier against dehydration, foreign bodies and UV radiation are now well established:

> Continued basic science and clinical research coupled with keen clinical observation has led to more recent recognition and general acceptance that the stratum corneum completes many vital 'barrier' tasks, including but not limited to regulating epidermal water content and the magnitude of water loss; mitigating exogenous oxidants that can damage components of skin via an innate antioxidant system; preventing or limiting cutaneous infection via multiple antimicrobial peptides; responding via innate immune mechanisms to 'cutaneous invaders' of many origins, including microbes, true allergens, and other antigens; and protecting its neighboring cutaneous cells and structures that lie beneath from damaging effects of ultraviolet radiation. (Del Rosso and Levin 2011, p.22)

It is clear that it is preferable for this layer of skin to remain intact, which is not the case in ablative therapies, which smooth out fine lines and scars by removing the epidermis and injuring the dermis. The downside is that these more invasive techniques result in a thinner epidermis being formed with less protection than before. This means that the skin is more vulnerable to the factors that lead to the reduction of collagen originally.

There is, of course, a place for ablative treatments, such as for hyperpigmentation, tattoo removal and acne reduction. Although skin needling is, in my view, a more effective way of reducing scars and treating ageing skin, MNT is particularly effective for improving acne scarring:

> Overall 36 out of the total of 37 patients completed the treatment schedule and were evaluated for its efficacy. Out of these 36 patients, 34 achieved a reduction in the severity of their scarring by one or two grades. More than 80% of patients assessed their treatment as 'excellent' on a 10-point scale. No significant adverse effects were noted in any patient. (Majid 2009, p.26)

Also, a study entitled 'Acne Scarring Treatment Using Skin Needling' published in 2008 had similar findings. Notably, all 32 patients who undertook the study had smoother skin after eight weeks following only the first treatment and it was concluded that the 'reduction in severity grade of acne scars before and after CIT, should be considered significant' (Fabbrocini *et al.* 2009, p.878).

The wound healing process is complex, but Fabbrocini *et al.* (2009) go on to discuss a new hypothesis that skin needling with a high-quality device does not 'create a wound in the classic sense'; however, 'the final result is a deposition of new collagen in the upper dermis'. This summary explains the concept more fully:

> The wound healing process is cut short, as the body is somehow 'fooled' into believing that an injury has occurred. According to this new theory, bioelectricity (also called 'demarcation current') triggers a cascade of growth factors that stimulate the healing phase. When microneedles penetrate the skin, they cause fine wounds. Cells react to this intrusion with a demarcation current that is additionally

increased by the needles' own electrical potential. (Fabbrocini
et al. 2009, p.878)

So, in short, collagen is produced in the dermis at various stages of the
healing process and continues to be laid down in the weeks and months
ahead. This natural process has the effect of plumping out facial scars and
fine lines and wrinkles, as well as helping to shrink the pores. This all occurs
without damaging the protective barrier of the outer layer of skin, making
it, to my mind, a preferable cosmetic procedure to more invasive methods.

The second key benefit of Micro Needle Therapy is the dramatic increase
in absorption of topically applied creams. The micro needles temporarily
open up miniscule channels, allowing serums and creams to by-pass the
barrier properties of the *stratum corneum* and penetrate to the underlying
dermis. This is one of the main advantages of the treatment; however, it
greatly demonstrates why we need to ensure the use of only high-quality,
professional topical products following needling, whether for MNT or
Facial Enhancement Acupuncture.

CHAPTER 6

TREATING SPECIFIC
FACIAL ISSUES

The main Facial Enhancement Acupuncture protocol will suffice for most facial issues, as it is working on a number of levels. However, should you wish to add to this to optimise the improvement of specific conditions, I have included some follow-up points that can be used.

First, let us take another look at the meridians of the body and how they relate to the face.

6.1 THE ACUPUNCTURE MERIDIANS AND THEIR ROLE IN FACIAL ENHANCEMENT ACUPUNCTURE

REN CHANNEL

- Regulates the body's Yin energy.

- Used to treat lifelessness in the face.

DU CHANNEL

- Regulates the body's Yang energy.

- Helps to treat internal organ conditions.

- Reduces swelling.

- Clears heat.

LIVER CHANNEL

- Beneficial for the eyes.

- Liver Qi stagnation can cause facial discolouration, dark circles and age spots.

GALL BLADDER CHANNEL

- Works with the Liver meridian to promote Qi and blood flow to the face.

HEART CHANNEL

- Excess Heart Fire can result in facial redness.

- A dull complexion can relate to Heart deficiency.

- Houses the *Shen*; relates to emotions, calms the mind, improves sleep, lessens stress and anxiety, all of which can lead to better skin.

SMALL INTESTINE CHANNEL

- Imbalance can lead to impurities manifesting (e.g. acne).

PERICARDIUM CHANNEL

- Protects the Heart.

TRIPLE HEATER

- 'The upper burner distributes fluids as a vapour over the entire body – it moistens the skin' (Hecker *et al.* 2005, p.247).

STOMACH CHANNEL

- Packed full of Qi and Blood.
- Promotes healing.
- Smooth flow of Qi will reduce puffiness, swelling and oedema.

SPLEEN CHANNEL

- Transporter of food Essence and fluids; aids the facial muscles and complexion.

LUNG CHANNEL

- Governs the skin.
- Responsible for opening and closing of the pores.
- Useful for treating acne.

LARGE INTESTINE CHANNEL

- Responsible for fluids.
- Eliminates toxins.
- Important organ for skin quality.

BLADDER CHANNEL

- The longest meridian passing both head and face.

KIDNEY CHANNEL

- Responsible for the reproductive system.
- Used to treat signs of premature ageing.

6.2 SAGGING FACIAL MUSCLES

As we age, our skin loses its firmness and elasticity; this is evident in our physique, as well as facially. What do we do about it? Well, if we are keen, and able to stick at it, we exercise and go to the gym regularly to try to tighten up those sagging muscles. We need to do exactly the same for the face; this can be achieved with facial exercises or we can try Facial Enhancement Acupuncture. This treatment gives the muscles of the face a work-out and also simultaneously stimulates the Qi to help with circulation. The resulting production of collagen helps to bring back some elasticity into the face.

Many of the facial points in the protocol have been selected, in part, for their relation to the underlying muscles. If you have established that facial sagging is the main focus of the treatment, you may like to add in this 'propeller' technique on the cheek.

Needle size: 15mm (length) × 0,20mm (thickness)/36 (gauge).

Technique: In addition to the Cheek Point used in the protocol, choose an *ashi* point on the cheek. An *ashi* point is an unnamed acupuncture point chosen for its sensitivity and location. Palpate to find an area where you can feel the band of muscle running across the cheekbone. Insert the needle into the point and twirl the needle in a clockwise direction, but with an action similar to winding up a propeller on a rubber-band aircraft. What we are attempting to do is to catch the facial muscle with the needle and tighten it with the twirling action. If this technique is administered successfully, you should find a lot of tension on the needle as you do this. Needle this point bilaterally. To remove the needle, it is a case of pulling back on the needle and gently unwinding the needle in an anti-clockwise direction; it can then be safely removed.

If you have a patient with significant facial sagging, it might be appropriate to use two or three of the skin tightening points on either side of the face.

6.3 EYE BAGS AND DARK CIRCLES

When we are treating a patient's eyes and the surrounding area, we also need to look at the constitutional points that we might be able to use in order to improve the appearance. Many patients come to me complaining of eye bags and a general puffiness under the eye. According to Traditional Chinese Medicine (TCM), all diseases that relate to the eye are closely linked to the Liver, as this meridian opens at the eyes. In Five Element Acupuncture, the Liver is the organ that is responsible for the smooth flow of Blood and Qi in the body. If this organ is out of balance, then there is a very good chance your patient will be stuck, perhaps congested and unable to move freely. This might, in my opinion, result in stagnation and consequential dark circles around the eye. In order to release this congestion and have the Qi flowing smoothly again, I would look at treating the Liver Source point LV3. This is a point that we are already using in our Initial Grounding Treatment as part of the Four Gates treatment, alongside LI4. I would pay particular attention to these points and tonify them at the end of the treatment, as LI4 will further help to reduce any swelling or oedema.

The partner organ of the Liver is the Gall Bladder and both meridians are of the Wood Element. One of my favourite Gall Bladder points for anything eye-related is GB41 'Foot Above Tears'. What a perfect name, which sums up exactly what it can do. Already in use as part of the main protocol, this in combination with LV3 is recommended for anything that involves stagnation of the eye.

ST44 is one of the first points that we needle and it is a great point to help clear stagnation. If it is immediately apparent on your first consultation that this eye condition is of concern to your patient, then I would definitely not omit ST44 from your Initial Grounding Treatment.

Bluish eye bags can be a sign that the Kidney channel is affected and fluid is being retained. KI3 is a Shu Stream point, and these 'points of the Yin channels are the primary point on each channel for regulating and harmonising their respective zang, and may therefore be considered as the single most important point of their respective channel' (Deadman 1993, p.36).

BL1 has to be needled slowly and with extreme caution, due to its location, but it can aid with fluid retension around the eye and other eye issues.

We already use ST2 during the protocol and this will help to reduce swelling to the lower eye by moving Qi and Blood to the area. Auricular points that can be added are, of course, the Eye and also Spleen for its role as the transporter of fluids.

6.4 AGE SPOTS AND SKIN DISCOLOURATION

'Surrounding the Dragon' is a technique that can be used for treating age spots and patches of hyperpigmentation. I absolutely love the description of this treatment; it actually sums up what we are trying to achieve so descriptively. Using 6mm intradermal needles, insert them so that they point towards the age spots/discolouration. The number of needles will vary, depending on the size of the target area, so you will need to use your judgement here. The main priority is to ensure that the area is completely surrounded. These needles can then be left in for the duration of the treatment and removed along with the other facial needles.

This technique helps fade age spots or discolouration by encircling the area with needles and thus redirecting the Qi underneath the damaged tissue, often caused by sun exposure, and ultimately outwards in a bid to regenerate the skin.

6.5 ACNE

Acne affects millions of people worldwide and is considered to be 'the most common cutaneous disorder in the Western World' (Goldberg and Berlin 2012, p.8). If someone presents with acne, I would generally begin with a course of Five Element Acupuncture treatment. However, there are general points that you could try to improve the condition based on Traditional Chinese Medicine principles. Acne is often attributed to the Lung–Large Intestine channels and the Spleen–Stomach channels. We have touched upon the subject of acne in earlier chapters and explored how the point ST9 could be utilised to treat overactive sebaceous glands (see Section 3.9) and how the application of pantothenic acid serum could improve acne and open pores (see Section 4.3.12). Retinol serum could also be applied to the skin. As it has a drying effect, however, care needs to be taken when using vitamin A. It should not be administered to those taking prescribed acne medication or anyone who is trying to conceive, is already pregnant or breast-feeding.

When the acne is caused by a hormonal imbalance, perhaps exacerbated during the menstrual cycle, the Endocrine auricular point can be used to help to balance the system. We have established the connection of the Lung meridian in connection with the skin, so I would also consider using LU5, a He-Sea point on the arm and the He-Sea point of the Large Intestine LI11, for its widely known benefits for skin issues.

The Spleen governs digestion and transportation, so stagnation in this channel may result in blemishes. Consider using the Spleen point on the ear to help the free flow of Qi along this meridian.

It is also possible to locate points around the infected area using the 'Surrounding the Dragon' technique outlined in Section 6.4.

6.6 ECZEMA

This dry skin condition, also known as dermatitis, is characterised by red, scaly and itchy skin that can vary in severity from person to person, especially as it comes in many different forms: 'In many developed countries over one-fifth of the population are affected by one or more atopic allergic disorders' (Sheikh 2002, p.14).

The skin of an eczema sufferer doesn't produce as much oil or fat as those without the condition. This lack of protection sees channels opening up because of the inability of the skin to retain water.

As both a Classical Five Element Acupuncturist and Facial Enhancement Acupuncturist, I am often called on to help with eczema on the body and I have also found that facial eczema can be particularly distressing to patients. The premise behind both traditional and facial acupuncture is that it is holistic, so we are aiming to balance Mind, Body and Spirit in order to help settle the problem. I would therefore tend to treat constitutional body points, before I begin to target specific areas.

I believe that how we look is very much related to how we feel, and eczema can be particularly debilitating due to the accompanying itch, which can be quite painful and lead to the skin splitting and bleeding. I would certainly suggest that a patient visit their doctor or dermatologist, particularly if their condition has yet to be diagnosed. What is very encouraging is that recent studies, such as 'Effect of Acupuncture on Allergen-Induced Basophil Activation in Patients with Atopic Eczema: A Pilot Trial' by Pfab *et al.* (2011), have been examining the successful reduction of itch intensity following treatment with acupuncture.

Apart from BL6 and BL2 on the head and face and the AE Drain that we can choose to perform at the patient's first treatment, we do not use any other Bladder points during the treatment. This is due to the fact that, as the meridian runs down the back and the back of the legs, it is not an easy channel to access whilst your patient is having facial acupuncture. However, there are a couple of points that may be worth tonifying at the start of treatment in this case. BL17 on the back and BL40, a He-Sea point on the back of the leg, are commonly used for itching skin.

'Family studies say that atopic disorders result from a complex interplay between genetic and environmental factors' (Sheikh 2002, p.16). And, like many conditions, the triggers can vary, so diet may be a factor or stress may result in a flare-up. Your patients may also find that climate could play a part or household allergies. Stress seems to be a common trigger for many of my patients and they find that the acupuncture helps in this regard. There have been many studies carried out that highlight the role acupuncture can play in reducing anxiety and one, albeit small, study, focusing on a single acupuncture point H7 (Shen Men), found an average 44 per cent reduction in stress (Chan *et al.* 2002, p.74). The Shen Men auricular point is needled bilaterally every treatment and this could be used to garner the same effects.

The Facial Enhancement Acupuncture protocol will aid with general inflammation and swelling as many of the points included are indicated for this. Again, I would suggest LU5 and LI11 could be tried for their relation to skin conditions.

6.7 ROSACEA

Rosacea is characterised by 'two clinical components: a vascular change consisting of intermittent or persistent erythema and flushing and an acneiform eruption with papules, pustules, cysts, and sebaceous hyperplasia' (Arndt and Hsu 2007, p.174). If you are a sufferer, or you have treated patients with rosacea in your own practice, you will know how this chronic skin condition can affect self-esteem and confidence.

Often, rosacea strikes in middle-age, as redness on the nose, cheeks, forehead and chin. Patients will experience different triggers and the most common seems to be sun exposure, closely followed by emotional stress. As practitioners, we regularly advise on lifestyle factors, so it is worth your patient trying to determine what may be exacerbating the condition.

We can help to balance the Body, Mind and Spirit and, as for other skin conditions, I would focus on my Five Element Acupuncture training to help address this issue. That said, I have had good success with rosacea from my Facial Enhancement Acupuncture protocol alone, as I find that it really activates the Qi in the face and helps to clear the skin. Depending on your patient's response to the initial protocol, LU5 and LI11 could also be added to your treatment plan to see if this boosts the effects.

If your patient has already established their triggers, it is important to find out whether they may be related to any of the creams you choose to use during a facial treatment. That is another reason for sourcing cleansers, serums and post-treatment creams that are beneficial and suitable for sensitive skin.

With four subtypes of rosacea (Erythematotelangiectatic, Papulopustular, Phymatous and Ocular), it is important to take your usual in-depth consultation and to discuss the realistic expectations about the outcomes of treatment depending upon their particular condition. The beauty of acupuncture is that it accepts that everyone is different and ensures that we maintain the holistic experience that this truly wonderful practice provides.

CHAPTER 7

FACIAL ENHANCEMENT ACUPUNCTURE CASE STUDIES

7.1 CASE STUDY 1: JANE, AGED 58

This case study that I would like to share with you is for one of my first Facial Enhancement patients. Jane came to me when she was in her late fifties, married with no children. A typical middle-aged lady, Jane was experiencing a few difficulties in life and wanting to get rid of some of the lines that had appeared over the years.

When we first talked, I could see that there was a lot more to Jane than just someone who wanted to try to turn back the clock; things went a lot deeper than that. I could tell there were issues of self-worth and also self-esteem that went back many years. During that initial consultation, it became obvious to me that this lady needed more help than just getting rid of a few of those lines.

You may be reading this and thinking, 'What has this got to do with facial acupuncture and helping reduce the signs of ageing?' Well, at this stage, not a great deal. However, as we go into greater detail, I hope that you will see the relevance of this case study in the context of facial acupuncture.

Jane had not experienced an acupuncture treatment before and was relatively new to alternative therapies in general. There was a very deep sadness to Jane that would take some time to get to the bottom of and, I hoped, help with. We carried on with our initial consultation and discussed the reasons why she had sought out cosmetic acupuncture as a treatment. It emerged that Jane had been unhappy about how she looked for quite a long while. I asked her to describe how she saw herself and what she would like to improve, if she could.

If we analyse how Jane looked, we can then consider how we might be able to help using Facial Enhancement Acupuncture. Her skin quality was reasonably good, with no visible oily patches or dry areas. She did have a lot of lines around the corners of the mouth and also on the top lip. Also evident was a loss of muscle structure around the mouth and chin, which gave the impression of a sagging mouth with deep lines vertically at the sides.

There was very little evidence of lines around the eyes and the 'number elevens', above the nose, were not too deep. There were a few furrows across the forehead, but again these were not that pronounced.

Generally, for a woman in her late fifties, Jane looked very good, perhaps just showing the usual signs of ageing. My overall impression, though, was still of this deep sadness and a general greyish colour to the whole face.

I decided that the best course of action would be a few Five Element Acupuncture treatments before we embarked on a course of Facial Enhancement Acupuncture. This was definitely a good plan, as it later emerged that Jane had gone through, and was still going through, quite a few personal difficulties. I was sure that we would be able to help with a course of acupuncture.

Let us fast-forward a couple of months. In a nutshell, I had established that Jane's Causative Factor (CF) was Metal. There was a lot of grief there and she was struggling to let go of things. Following ten acupuncture treatments working with her on all levels, both physically and emotionally, I was so glad that we decided to take this option. The sadness that was apparent at our first meeting had started to subside and the pallid colour had begun to lift. I felt that we were in a much better position now to embark on a series of Facial Enhancement Acupuncture treatments.

We had talked earlier about the patient's lack of muscle tone around the mouth. This is a very difficult area to improve dramatically, as the face has a pronounced sunken look to it after that amount of muscle wastage. We planned an initial course of ten Facial Enhancement Acupuncture treatments at weekly intervals, followed by regular maintenance treatment every six to eight weeks.

The patient responded really positively to the facial treatments, especially as she had experienced Five Element treatment and was feeling a great deal better after her course of regular acupuncture. Consequently, the Facial Enhancement Acupuncture treatments went very well and there did seem to be a marked improvement in the general appearance of the skin; the fine lines across the forehead were also reduced. As I first thought and explained to the patient, it was difficult to make a marked impression in the area around the mouth, but there did seem to be an improvement in the fullness of the face there and the patient was very pleased with the results.

Jane was a perfect example of a Facial Enhancement Acupuncture patient who needed a little bit more than just cosmetic treatment, and in the end I was really pleased to be able to help her on so many levels, other than just her appearance. To this day, Jane is still a regular patient at my clinic and she continues to have monthly Five Element Acupuncture treatments, plus a Facial Enhancement Acupuncture treatment every couple of months. Over the period of time that she has been having these treatments, she still feels that there are improvements to her face. She is a great fan of the treatment and, most importantly, she feels better too.

7.2 CASE STUDY 2: PETRA, AGED 35

Petra is a young lady who came to me a couple of years ago wanting help with her acne.

My first impressions of her complaint were that it did not seem too severe but, obviously, when something is of concern to the individual, then in their eyes it sometimes seems more problematic than it actually might be.

Generally, her skin looked to be in very good condition; the main problem were the raised cheek areas that were showing some old acne scars and also some current spots that were very red.

After a traditional diagnosis, the first course of treatment was an Aggressive Energy Drain (see Section 3.1). This was used to balance the patient, before carrying out facial treatment.

Following the initial consultation, it was again decided to treat this patient's Metal Element. Therefore, I selected Lung and Large Intestine points as a constitutional treatment, alongside the Facial Enhancement Acupuncture protocol. This would help to eliminate any toxins that had built up in the system.

Note: This detoxification process could appear to exacerbate the problem for a few days, so it is important to explain that this may be the case, but reassure your patient that this will soon calm down.

A good way to treat a patient suffering with active acne would be to perform a treatment comprised of some additional constitutional points, combined with facial points. To begin with, I used a treatment called 'Surrounding the Dragon'; this is a treatment where we use acupuncture needles in *ashi* points circulating the offending area (see Section 6.4). I inserted the needles around the acne and not into the blemishes themselves and slightly angled towards the offending area.

The aim of this treatment is to promote healing to the skin that we are concentrating on, targeting the body's own healing energy into the condition. A noticeable improvement in the patient's acne condition was seen after three treatments. This was as a result of the constitutional treatment using the Metal points and also the 'Surrounding the Dragon' treatments.

Along with the additional treatment for the patient's acne, I also carried out the full Facial Enhancement Acupuncture protocol. Because this patient had existing acne scars from previous breakouts, it was decided that I would try to help to erase these marks by using intradermal needles directly into the scars. The aim of the treatment was to stimulate collagen production in the skin that was affected by the scarring and plump out the pitted scars.

Once the active acne was under control and after closer examination during the treatments, it was decided that the patient would benefit from Micro Needle Therapy (MNT) treatment using dermal rollers to help further reduce the acne scarring. The MNT has the same effect as the intradermals, but is ideal when there is a larger area to treat.

The results of the MNT treatment were dramatic and, after a couple of treatments, with six weeks in between, there was a significant reduction in the appearance of the scars.

7.3 SAMPLE CASE STUDIES

I have included a selection of short case studies based on a typical initial Facial Enhancement Acupuncture treatment. These are general outlines and even patients exhibiting the same facial issues will often vary in the type of treatment carried out and the expected results. Every individual is different and we must always bear this in mind when forming our treatment plan. These studies are here to provide a basic guideline as to how you can successfully tailor your treatments centred upon your patient's unique requirements.

PATIENT 1

Treatment focus: Forehead and mouth.

Techniques used: First, I used the grounding and anaesthesia points and followed with those on the cheek and jaw; the patient had pointed out that they wanted particular attention paid to the mouth area. I achieved a nice pulling and tucking effect with the use of point ST4 and the Extra points under the mandible bone. I then moved on to the points on the front of the face to include ST3 and SI18. Next, I used the 'Surrounding the Dragon' technique on the forehead around some age spots and areas of discolouration. The whole treatment was finished with a facial massage, paying particular attention to the forehead by using the Chinese Gua Sha technique

Expected results: Using the 'Surrounding the Dragon' technique on a regular basis should result in a distinct improvement in age spots.

PATIENT 2

Treatment focus: Vertical lines between the eyebrows and horizontal lines across the forehead. Moderately dry skin.

Techniques used: The treatment started with the grounding, as well as the anaesthesia, points. The patient complained of tension in her neck, so I included the points ST13 and GB21. The skin felt very taut when I needled the Cheek and Jaw points and I was able to get a good lift on the eyebrow area. All Face and Cheek points were inserted comfortably. I used the 'Surrounding the Dragon' points primarily on the forehead. The vertical lines between the eyebrows were treated with intradermal needles and this was also the case with the horizontal forehead lines. After the treatment I used hyaluronic acid on the whole face, but focusing on the vertical and horizontal lines.

Expected results: With continued treatment and the use of the hyaluronic acid, we should see a dramatic reduction in the intensity of the brow and forehead lines. The skin should also become less dry, due to the hydrating qualities of the hyaluronic acid.

PATIENT 3

Treatment focus: Red complexion.

Techniques used: I used the Four Gates and some cooling points to help with the patient's high blood pressure, LI11, LV2, DU20 and also ST9 later on. I then followed the full Facial Enhancement Acupuncture protocol. After I needled the legs and hand points, I decided to use Shen Men and Sympathetic auricular points. I worked on the eyebrow points and found this to be a sensitive area, so I think I will use numbing cream there for future treatments. I then moved on to the points on the front of the face. I used the intradermal needles on the only deep lines running from the nose to the corners of the mouth.

Expected results: ST9 is a useful point for taking heat and redness out of the face. After a few treatments you would expect the redness in the face start to subside.

PATIENT 4

Treatment focus: Dark pigmentation beneath the eyes.

Techniques used: For the grounding treatment I used Shen Men, ST44, LV3 and GB41. I added the Point Zero auricular point and then performed the full facial treatment protocol.

Expected results: Immediately after treatment, the patient's eyes should look a lot brighter. The use of Wood points, Liver and Gall Bladder will have a profound effect on the eyes.

PATIENT 5

Treatment focus: The skin is not overly wrinkled, but the patient complains of saggy jowls.

Techniques used: The patient's pulse was a little fast, and she said she gets anxious before any procedure. I began with the auricular points Shen Men and Point Zero and she soon began to relax. I used all of the points in a Facial Enhancement Acupuncture procedure, but made a conscious effort to really work on the points under the mandible bone. I added Mandible as a third auricular point to help strengthen this area.

Expected results: Needling the jaw area is a bit tricky at first, but with a little practice you can achieve a very tight area beneath the jaw line. With continued treatment there should be a dramatic improvement on the jowl area.

PATIENT 6

Treatment focus: Around the eyes.

Techniques used: This was a new patient, so to start this treatment protocol I first carried out an Aggressive Energy Drain. Following this I needled the Four Gates points. I moved on to the auricular points of Shen Men and the Eye point, followed by DU20 and BL6, and continued with the full Facial Enhancement Acupuncture protocol. I then inserted the intradermal needles at the eyebrows. I focused on the 'crow's feet', inserting intradermal needles on both sides at a spacing of a couple of millimetres. I then performed a Jade Roller Massage, placing specific emphasis on the eye area with the smaller roller.

Expected results: A patient's eyes are often noticeably better following Five Element Acupuncture but, following the full facial protocol, this is often amplified. After only one treatment, I regularly see a great improvement around the eyes, but also in the eyes themselves and in their clarity.

PATIENT 7

Treatment focus: This patient wanted me to focus on her cheeks and jaws and around her eyes where 'crow's feet' were forming. Her cheeks were somewhat red and beginning to lose firmness.

Techniques used: I needled the Four Gates, Shen Men and the auricular Cheek point. This time, I chose to needle the anaesthesia points PC4 and TH8, achieving *De-Qi*. The patient had very little experience of acupuncture and was concerned about the possibility of pain and discomfort. The combination of Shen Men and Yin Tang also helped the patient to feel very calm. The cheek was my focal point for this patient so I needled these points with an upward direction. After checking that the patient was comfortable, I moved on to the eye area, and used intradermal needles in the crow's feet. As usual, I left the intradermal needles in place for 20 minutes and after that I proceeded to carefully remove the needles, starting with intradermals and facial needles and ending up removing LV3 as the final needle.

Expected results: The cheeks may seem more red initially following treatment, but this should decrease and be replaced by a lighter complexion colour. The patient's cheeks should appear less swollen and the skin more taut.

PATIENT 8

Treatment focus: Normal to dehydrated skin, enlarged pores, brown spots. The patient also has wrinkles and fine lines in between the eyebrows, in the nasal labial fold and on the top lip.

Techniques used: I started as usual with an AE Drain, followed by the Four Gates point and continued with the other constitutional body points. The patient complained of very dehydrated skin. This should improve dramatically by using the Facial Enhancement Acupuncture protocol. I used the intradermal needles on the lines around the eyes and also along the nasal labial fold. Thirty minutes before needling the top lip lines, I decided to apply some skin-numbing cream as this particular area can be very sensitive. I applied hyaluronic acid, with pantothenic acid to lock in moisture and help to shrink the pores. There was a lot to focus on for the initial treatment and I will wait to see the developments before adding in the 'Surrounding the Dragon' method to tackle the age spots.

Expected results: There should be a dramatic improvement in skin quality, due to the increased circulation to the face. After only a few treatments there should be a great improvement on the lines around the eyes and the nasal labial fold.

PATIENT 9

Treatment focus: This patient has been having Botox® for 'crow's feet' and 'number elevens'. The appointment was scheduled three months following the patient's last Botox® session, as an alternative to having the more invasive treatments.

Techniques used: I made some diet and lifestyle recommendations as the patient had complained of general unhealthiness and diet issues. Many of the Facial Enhancement Acupuncture points can aid detox, such as LI4, LV3, GB41, ST36, SP9, Yin Tang and DU20. Alongside Shen Men, the auricular points I selected were Liver and Eye, and I added in Large Intestine to help the detoxification process. I focused on the areas that the patient had received Botox® for and also for eye bags. I also used intradermal needles in the 'number elevens' between the eyebrows and the 'crow's feet'. There was noticeable erythema in these areas following needling.

Expected results: A general softening of the lines on the face should occur but, because of the effects of the Botox®, it will take a few treatments to have any lasting result.

PATIENT 10

Treatment focus: Facial sagging, loose skin in the cheek and also around the jaw area.

Techniques used: I needled the constitutional body points and I chose to use a few more auricular points with this patient. Shen Men, of course, but also Mandible, Cheek and Spleen for its relation to the toning of the flesh. I used the 'propeller' technique described in Section 6.2, to help tighten up the cheek muscles and spent time using the 'pinning' method (see Section 4.3.7) to tighten the skin beneath the jaw.

Expected results: The patient should see an initial lifting effect after the first treatment, although they will need a few more sessions to really gain benefit from the treatment.

PATIENT 11

Treatment focus: Lines around the mouth.

Technique used: Because of the quantity of lines around the mouth, it was necessary to use in excess of 50 intradermals just in this one area.

Expected results: There should be some change within approximately three treatments, but I would also recommend introducing some sessions of Micro Needle Therapy every 4–6 weeks. Used in combination with regular FEA treatments, this should see dramatic results in this area.

PATIENT 12

Treatment focus: Overall complexion and forehead lines.

Techniques used: I needled the Four Gates and the body points, omitting the anaesthetic points as this was a regular patient who is not sensitive to needling. I then proceeded with the facial protocol. I used intradermal needles for the forehead lines and selected the Forehead auricular point. The overall complexion of the patient should naturally improve by the use of the Facial Enhancement Acupuncture protocol. The facial needles generate a lot of Qi and this is circulated throughout the face, resulting in an improvement in complexion and reducing open pores. I applied retinol serum to the face and used the Gua Sha stone to push it into the skin.

Expected results: The improved Qi energy and blood flow that the needling to the face promotes should see a rapid improvement to the complexion within approximately three treatments.

PATIENT 13

Treatment focus: Facial scar and active acne.

Techniques used: I carried out the full Facial Enhancement Acupuncture protocol. The patient had an old scar on her face and I used the 'Surrounding the Dragon' technique. I chose not to opt for Micro Needle Therapy to treat this, as the patient had active acne that needed addressing and this would not be recommended in relation to Dermal Rolling. In addition to this, I made sure that I needled ST9 and also selected LU5 and LI11 to help the skin. I applied hyaluronic acid serum, with pantothenic acid to help the infection.

Expected results: The 'Surrounding the Dragon' technique can significantly reduce the appearance of a scar over a period of approximately six treatments. The acne can get worse initially, due to the detoxification process. However, it should then begin to improve to the point where we can use MNT to further plump out the pitted scar.

PATIENT 14

Treatment focus: Old acne scars.

Techniques used: Whilst it was important to carry out a full Facial Enhancement Acupuncture treatment on this patient, it was also deemed beneficial to carry out a series of dermal roller treatments that would directly help to reduce the appearance of the acne scars.

Expected results: The dermal roller can be used as stand-alone treatment, but it is also a valuable tool when used in combination with the Facial Enhancement Acupuncture treatment. On this particular patient, it would be envisaged that a vast improvement would be evident after approximately six treatments, carried out at 4–6 week intervals.

PATIENT 15

Treatment focus: Sagging eyebrows and eyelids.

Techniques used: First, I carried out an Aggressive Energy Drain with this patient; this was followed by the Four Gates treatment. I decided to apply some numbing cream to the eyebrows as this area can be very sensitive. Once the numbing cream had taken effect, I needled points BL6, GB14 and the three intradermal points that lift the eyebrow. The rest of the Facial Enhancement Acupuncture protocol was carried out and the needles left in place for 20 minutes.

Expected results: An improvement to the eyebrows should be evident after approximately three treatments, which should also affect the eyelid. I would envisage that this would improve even more over a full course of ten treatments.

CHAPTER 8

MARKETING FACIAL ENHANCEMENT ACUPUNCTURE

The subject of marketing is something that is very close to my heart, having spent many years in a sales and marketing career before I discovered I was far happier sticking needles in people. Joking apart, this background did set me up with some knowledge of how I might be able to attract patients to my clinic and also, more importantly, keep them as regular patients in my practice.

My emphasis with marketing and patients has always been focused on patient retention. It is so important to make sure that your patients come back to you on a regular basis and that you have offers and services that will attract them. A very simple way to achieve this, and something that you might do already, is always to make sure that at the end of a patient's treatment you rebook them for a follow-up. This could be in a week or even three months' time. As long as you get a date booked in the diary, you can relax, as you know you will be seeing that patient again. There is nothing worse, in my mind, than a happy patient going away and saying they will be in touch or they will see how things get on. Of course, you cannot hold a patient down and not let them out until they rebook, but there is nothing stopping you having the diary ready and suggesting some dates. The other side of this issue is when you have a cancellation. There is nothing that can be done to change this, but when it happens, ensure that you try to get into the habit of making a new booking as soon as they cancel. If they telephone and leave a message, the same applies. It never does any harm to return the call or send an email expressing your concerns that they are okay and to suggest booking a date for their appointment in the future.

If, as a practitioner, you maintain constant contact with your patients and keep an efficient diary, you should always have a healthy and busy practice. We will review some of these tips later and organise them into some user-friendly reminders to help jog your memory.

Of course, the main idea behind this chapter is to help you market facial acupuncture and to bring prospective patients into your practice; the same methods and techniques can be used for any type of acupuncture or business. It is simply a case of tailoring them to suit your current need. Let us break down the subject of marketing into some bite-size chunks that we can take in more easily.

8.1 MARKETING TO EXISTING PATIENTS

This is probably the most overlooked but most accessible opportunity to add business to your practice. Think about every patient that you treat. Obviously they are happy with the service that you have given them; otherwise they would not be a regular patient. During the time that you have been seeing them you will have built up a sound knowledge of their background and personality. More importantly, they will trust your abilities and judgement. So, before you even start to think about an advertisement in the paper, start talking to your regulars. Ask them questions. Would they like to try a facial acupuncture treatment? Perhaps you might like to offer them a special discounted treatment as a thank you for being a loyal patient. Have some discount vouchers printed and give them to patients to pass on to friends and relatives. This is a good way to spread the word.

Another effective method of advertising to your regular patients is to organise an open day or evening where you will be demonstrating the new treatments and answering any questions about what you have to offer.

Remember old or lapsed patients; I am sure you have a filing cabinet of files for patients who have not been to your practice for a while. With a new treatment to offer, this provides a perfect opportunity to rekindle some interest and get them back in to see you. Of course, they may also have friends or relatives who may be keen to try acupuncture, so put together a professional letter along the lines of: 'It has been a while since we saw you at the clinic, so we would like to let you know about some exciting new developments that I am sure will be of interest.' Remember to include some discount vouchers too.

You can be very daring in your marketing to existing patients; it can take some bravery on your part, but it can also bring long-term dividends. Perhaps take a look at your patient database and list your top 50 regular patients. Then produce a card or email that thanks them for their continued support and offer them a free facial acupuncture treatment. There is a possibility that you may get a few joking responses: 'So you think I need something done with my face?' However, remember that anyone can benefit from Facial Enhancement Acupuncture, young or old, male or female. This type of marketing is extremely powerful; if we look at it more carefully, you are thanking one of your most loyal patients by offering them a free treatment. Depending on your treatment charges, this could be to the value of £100. Obviously, this free offer does not cost you this amount, but your patient does not see this; they only see the free £100 treatment.

It might go against your business ideals to be giving away treatments, but do not look at it as giving something away; look at it as an investment in your new business. These 50 patients are the core of your business; they will spread the word and, more importantly, they will rebook if they like the treatment that you provide.

And that brings me nicely into the next step of using your existing patient base to its full. Introduce a 'refer a friend' scheme. You could set up a system that rewards your patients when they introduce a new patient to your clinic – perhaps a discount off of their next treatment for every new patient they introduce. Printing some referral cards can be a simple and effective way of marketing your practice.

Whilst you are having these printed, you could also opt to produce some patient loyalty cards. These are a great way to retain your patients and also introduce them to your new treatments. One suggestion might be to stamp the patient's card every time they have a treatment and then, as a bonus, the tenth treatment could be a free facial acupuncture treatment. This is a great way of keeping your patients loyal and also thanking them for their continued custom.

8.2 ATTRACTING NEW PATIENTS

This section is particularly relevant to practitioners just starting out, but can apply to anyone seeing a dip in trade or for general maintenance of your diary.

There are so many ways that you can attract new patients to your clinic; the main thing is to think about who you are trying to attract and not to waste money on general advertising that, in my experience, very rarely works. When thinking of Facial Enhancement Acupuncture, a certain client stream will initially come to mind. Who might like to try facial acupuncture, perhaps as an alternative to other facial procedures? Approach a few local hairdressers in your area – see if they might be interested in advertising your facial treatments to their clients. You can reward them for displaying your leaflets, perhaps with a commission for anyone they send your way. They might even like the idea of you doing a demonstration evening for their clients. Further down the line, you may even find an establishment with a spare room that you could rent on a regular basis and offer onsite treatments directly to their clients.

Obviously, facial acupuncture is for both sexes, but of course it is only natural that it is going to appeal to women more than men. Do some research into groups and organisations in your area that cater mainly for women; these could be organisations like the Women's Institute or other groups that meet on a regular basis. I have found that groups such as these are always looking for speakers at their meetings and this is a great opportunity to gather 20 or 30 women in one place to talk about your subject.

The prospect of talking to a hall of 30 people might not be for you, but try not to dismiss the idea too quickly. In general, they will only require you to speak for 30–45 minutes and that is not too long to talk about a subject that you are knowledgeable and passionate about. From my experience, you do not need any fancy props or projectors. I simply take along a few needles so that I can dispel the myths and then I talk about acupuncture and how it can help. I then let the audience ask a few questions and before you know it nearly an hour has passed. Make sure you have plenty of leaflets on hand and also take along your diary, as some people will want to book an appointment there and then – make sure you are ready to take those bookings.

Leaflet drops are another way of getting the word out. In my experience, they are generally more successful than newspaper advertising, but not as good as regular talks and more direct marketing. Leafleting can get the word out very quickly, but do not expect a huge response. The odds are very low when it comes to this type of marketing; I usually look at perhaps a 2 per cent response rate. So, for every thousand leaflets, I would expect to get 20 new patients. However, by making your leaflets more attractive and aiming them at a specific sector of the public, this should help to improve the take-up odds. It is also important to have a clear 'call to action' on your flyer, perhaps with a code so that you know exactly how successful your campaign has been. A well-designed, targeted leaflet, with an offer, is more likely to be pinned to a noticeboard or fridge, rather than finding its way straight to the dustbin.

Leafleting should be part of an overall marketing campaign and should not be your sole method of attaining new business. Coupled with other forms of direct marketing, it can be a powerful tool to build your brand locally.

We should not overlook other forms of media, such as local radio and, of course, television. The latter can be difficult to get on to, but local radio is a very realistic option for your marketing. We all have nearby stations that may be interested in hearing from you. They all have time spots to fill and would be really interested to hear about what you do. Of course, you cannot just use the radio to advertise, unless you pay for airtime, but what you can do is use any airtime that you do get to spread the word and create awareness of what you are offering.

An effective way of introducing yourself to radio stations and also getting free coverage in newspapers is to produce a press release. A press release is a simple and concise document that informs the reader of something new and/or something that they might find interesting. There are many websites that can help you to produce a press release and it really is a worthwhile thing to do. Journalists are always on the lookout for items with a difference or that have relevance to topics in the national news. By sending your press release to the radio stations and also local newspapers, this could achieve airtime or editorial that could be worth a lot more than some paid advertising.

People like to hear from and deal with experts in their field and, after all, that is what you are. You have trained for years to do what you do and continue to gain experience treating your patients in your clinic. As well as the talks and lectures to groups, you might also like to consider writing short pieces for local magazines and community newspapers. Again, this is not a direct form of advertising, but a way of drip-feeding awareness to people and letting them know what you are offering and where they can go to benefit from your expertise.

8.3 ONLINE MARKETING

The benefit of being in practice these days is the access we all have to the internet and social media. We can communicate with hundreds if not thousands of potential new patients at the click of a button.

As a basic requirement, I would recommend that every practice has its own website, even if it is only a basic one-page site that you can add to as the practice grows. Make sure that your website tells people exactly what you do and where they can find you. You also need to ensure that your contact details are clear and easy to see, so that potential patients can readily book an appointment to see you. This may sound obvious, but it is surprising the number of websites I have come across that have not considered this. Also, your website should be a place of information and not just somewhere to advertise your business. You want visitors to keep coming back to your site on a regular basis and they will only do this if the site is interesting and offering new information. Nothing is worse than an old site that displays the same material; it is beneficial to keep the site as fresh as you can.

Make sure your website address is displayed on all of your literature and business cards; it needs to become the focus of your business – the place that tells people what is happening and keeps them updated with the latest developments. You could also incorporate or link your own blog page to your website. I am sure you are familiar with blogs and may already write your own but, for those who are not, a blog is where you write about a variety of topics online. Subjects could be acupuncture or yourself, right through to developments in your clinic or the services that you offer. Again, it is more of a tool to provide information and resources than a direct sales aid, but it will help to develop and build your profile, which can direct business to your practice.

There is a vast array of social media avenues to explore, too many to mention here. For my clinic, I predominantly use Facebook, Twitter and LinkedIn. We have gradually gained a good following on Facebook and our Twitter account is linked to this. Social media can be time-consuming to maintain, but it is also very immediate and gets your message in front of an audience that has chosen to connect with you. This provides a distinct advantage over other types of marketing. As long as you are using it to engage with your community rather than solely to promote your business, I believe it can be a great addition to your marketing strategy. My advice would be to aim most of your posts at providing information and resources to your audience, rather than direct selling.

One of the most rewarding benefits of your website or social media platform is to gather information about your existing patients and also potential new patients for your clinic. Make sure that every visitor to your website or Facebook page has the opportunity to leave their email address as a minimum; also let them know that by leaving their details you would like to keep them informed of your services and any special deals that you might be offering. By making it clear to visitors that it is your intention to send updates and news about your business, you should not have any problems in using the information that you collect for marketing to this database.

One of the best ways of doing this is to produce a newsletter, perhaps monthly or quarterly. Use this as a chance to tell potential patients what has been happening at the clinic and any exciting new developments that are occuring. Of course, remember to provide your readers with resources and information. It is not all about selling. Your newsletter should be giving people information of value that they find interesting, that they want to share with their friends. It should be engaging, so that your audience will want to read more and receive future issues.

You may wish to provide an incentive to encourage people to sign up to your newsletter, such as a free guide, ebook or some top tips related to health and wellbeing that you have written. Many of the email marketing companies have a facility for automated emails that can be sent out when someone chooses to add themselves to your mailing list.

8.4 MEMBERSHIPS

It is all well and good having a brilliant website and engaging social media communities, but how do people find you in the first place? An effective website will have search engine optimisation in place and will climb to the first page of Google or other well-known search engines for relevant terms. You can also set up pay-per-click advertising campaigns that will direct people to your website or within Facebook, for example. This can be an effective method of promoting your online presence, but you will need to have a realistic budget in place and regularly quantify the results to get the best out of your campaigns. However, some people will still prefer to find practitioners through a trusted network or professional body and will look to these registers to find a qualified practitioner first.

As a traditional acupuncturist based in the UK, I am a member of the British Acupuncture Council and potential patients can find me through their website. You may practise Western medical acupuncture or auricular acupuncture or you may be a physiotherapist who has undertaken training in acupuncture. Each of these modalities will have their own societies or regulating bodies and I have listed some of those that are located in the UK in the resources section.

Membership of a site pertaining to your training can lend weight to your profile and reassures potential patients of your qualifications. There is a cost involved, and some of my colleagues have chosen to opt out of such groups, but from a personal perspective I have found membership to be beneficial to my practice. One of the major assets of these associations is that they provide a hub of information about the service that you are offering, building awareness of what you practise and enabling potential patients to discover more about acupuncture and how it can help them. The member areas also often provide the opportunity to talk with fellow practitioners about your business and the profession as a whole.

In the UK, there is now a network specifically for facial acupuncture and Micro Needle Therapy. I recognised that there was a gap in the market for acupuncturists specialising in this type of treatment and, in 2008, I founded Cosmetic Acupuncture UK. This professional network is open to acupuncture practitioners who have undergone additional training in cosmetic acupuncture. A sister-site for Five Element Acupuncturists, The 5 Element Acupuncture Network, was created in 2012 (see Resources).

Making your website available on these sites, and other related directories, not only links potential practitioners straight to your business but also helps your website's rank in the search engines, as they favour highly relevant backlinks.

8.5 BRANDING

The best way to bring all of these marketing ideas together, especially the website and the social media aspects, is to develop a brand for your business. A branding gives your business an identity that potential patients can recognise and relate to.

Branding covers everything from your business logo, through to the colours that you use on your printed literature and website. Your logo is important, but it does not need to be anything too grand; it might even just be your own name written in a style and colour that people will remember. The key is to create a uniform look that flows through all of your stationery, such as your business cards, flyers, letter head and advertising. This should then tie into your online presence, which will give a look and feel that endorses your professional skills. Good branding will give potential patients confidence in you and how you operate.

With any of these ideas that I have put forward, there is no need to employ expensive companies to develop things. Of course, you can invest in this if you choose, but these ideas can also be implemented by the individual. With a little thought and imagination, you will be able to put forward a brand and image that you can be proud of.

8.6 TOP TEN MARKETING TIPS FOR FACIAL ENHANCEMENT ACUPUNCTURE

The tips and ideas that I have outlined to help with the development of your new facial acupuncture business are simple but, when put together, can be very powerful at attracting new business. The ideas can be used in whole or in part, but my advice would be to employ as many of the suggestions as possible. If you do that, I can almost guarantee that you will have a full diary now and into the future.

I have broken my marketing tips down into a few easy stages below that summarise the suggestions that I have made. Some options will depend on your budget, but many simply need an investment of your time. In that respect, there is absolutely nothing to lose by giving some of these ideas a try and I am sure that you will be pleased by the results that can be achieved.

1. Introduce a 'refer a friend' scheme or loyalty card for existing patients.

2. Run a clinic open evening to introduce facial acupuncture.

3. Carry out a targeted leaflet drop for facial acupuncture.

4. Approach local groups to do talks.

5. Produce a facial acupuncture press release and send it to local radio, newspapers and magazines.

6. Develop or improve your website.

7. Set up social media accounts, such as Facebook and Twitter.

8. Look into adding your contact details to relevant online directories or becoming a member of a professional body, network, society or association.

9. Start a practice newsletter.

10. Develop your practice branding.

GLOSSARY

ACUPUNCTURE: An ancient Chinese treatment/medical technique based on the principle that there are pathways called meridians relating to internal organs and systems, running throughout the body. Vital energy or Qi flows along the meridian lines and there are points along these channels that can be stimulated by the insertion of fine sterile, disposable needles to clear blockages. Points are selected for the treatment of various disorders or to alleviate pain.

AGGRESSIVE ENERGY DRAIN: Treatment protocol used to clear an accumulation of unhealthy Qi energy from a patient's system.

ANAESTHESIA: Loss of bodily sensation, specifically loss of the feeling of pain.

ANALGESIA: An inability to feel pain.

ASHI POINT: Tender spots that can be used as acupuncture points.

AURICULAR: Relating to the ears.

BLOOD: Dense fluid that has been affected by Qi energy, flowing both through the vessels and the meridians, nourishing Body, Mind and Spirit.

BODY, MIND AND SPIRIT: If one of these three connecting factors is out of balance, it can affect the others.

CHANNELS: See 'Meridians'.

CUN MEASUREMENT: A Chinese measurement denoted by the width of the knuckle of the thumb or the space in between the distal and proximal inter-phalangeal joints of the third finger. 1.5 cun is measured by the width of first and second fingers together. All four fingers together demarcates 3 cun.

DE-QI: The sensation felt when stimulating an acupuncture point.

EVENS TECHNIQUE: Method where the acupuncture needle is inserted with no stimulation.

EXTRA POINT: Extraordinary acupuncture point that is not attributed to a particular channel.

HE-SEA POINT: Connecting points found at the elbows and knees.

INTRADERMAL NEEDLE: Small 3mm or 6mm acupuncture needle used for fine work.

JING: The Essence. Kidney *Jing*, derived from both pre- and post-Heaven Essence, is related to growth and maturation.

MERIDIANS: Channels of energy that run throughout the body.

QI: Vital energy believed to circulate around the body in currents.

SHEN: The Spirit. Heart *Shen* governs the emotions.

SHU-STREAM POINT: Where Qi pours through the channel.

SOURCE POINT: A high-concentration point that provides access to the main meridian system.

TCM: Traditional Chinese Medicine.

TONIFICATION: Stimulation of the acupuncture point by turning the needle clockwise to boost it.

XI-CLEFT POINT: Where Qi and Blood gather.

YING SPRING POINT: Acupuncture point where the Qi trickles down the meridian.

RESOURCES

www.facialenhance.co.uk
Facial Enhance, the home of Facial Enhancement Acupuncture, providing information, latest developments and details of upcoming masterclasses and workshops.

www.learncosmeticacupuncture.com
Facial Enhance online courses, including Facial Enhancement Acupuncture, Micro Needle Therapy and jade roller study options. Paul Adkins' training options including comprehensive study material and HD videos, resulting in certification and a listing as a practitioner on the Facial Enhance website.

www.cosmeticacupunctureuk.com
Cosmetic Acupuncture UK Network.

www.5Elementacupuncture.co.uk
The 5 Element Acupuncture Network.

www.acupuncture.org.uk
British Acupuncture Council, the UK's main regulatory body for the practice of traditional acupuncture

www.bawma.co.uk
British Academy of Western Medical Acupuncture, training medical doctors and nurses to practise Western medical acupuncture.

www.medical-acupuncture.co.uk
The British Medical Acupuncture Society. Western medical training for healthcare practitioners.

www.aacp.uk.com
Acupuncture Association of Chartered Physiotherapists.

www.auricularacupuncturecollege.com
The college of Auricular Acupuncture. Ear acupuncture study options.

www.facebook.com/facialenhancementacupuncture
Facebook page for Facial Enhance.

www.twitter.com/facialenhance
Twitter page for Facial Enhance.

www.5elementwebdesign.co.uk
Website design for therapists.

REFERENCES

Adkins, P. (2006) *The Pocket Guide to Facial Enhancement Acupuncture*. Raleigh, NC: Lulu.

Anon. (1974) *The Principles and Practical Use of Acupuncture Anaesthesia*. Hong Kong: Medicine & Health Publishing Co.

Anon. (1975) *Acupuncture Anesthesia*. Washington, DC: U.S. Department of Health, Education and Welfare.

Anon. (1991) *Sport Diving: The British Sub-Aqua Club Diving Manual*. London: Hutchinson.

Arndt, K.A. and Hsu, J.T.S. (2007) *Manual of Dermatologic Therapeutics*. Philadelphia, PA: Lippincott Williams & Wilkins.

Aust, M.C., Fernandes, D., Kolokythas, P., Kaplan, H.M. and Vogt, P.M. (2008) 'Percutaneous Collagen Induction Therapy: An Alternative Treatment for Scars, Wrinkles, and Skin Laxity.' *Plastic and Reconstructive Surgery 121*, 4, 1421–1429.

Barbano, R. (2006) 'Risks of Erasing Wrinkles: Buyer Beware!' *Neurology 67*, E17–E18.

Benedetto, A.V. (1999) 'The Cosmetic Uses of Botulinum Toxin Type A.' *International Journal of Dermatology 38*, 9, 641–655.

Birrell, A. (1999) *The Classic of Mountains and Seas*. Harmondsworth: Penguin Books.

Chan, J., Briscomb, D., Waterhouse, E. and Cannaby, A.-M. (2002) 'An Uncontrolled Pilot Study of HT7 for "Stress".' *Acupuncture in Medicine 20*, 2–3, 74–77.

Chen, P. (2004) *Modern Chinese Ear Acupuncture*. Taos, NM: Paradigm Publications.

Connelly, D.M. (1975) *Traditional Acupuncture: The Law of the Five Elements*. Columbia, NY: Centre for Traditional Acupuncture.

Deadman, P. (1993) 'The Five-Shu Points.' *Journal of Chinese Medicine 42*, 31–38.

Deadman, P. and Al-Khafaji, M. (1993) 'A Brief Discussion of the Points of the Window of Heaven.' *Journal of Chinese Medicine 43*, 32–34.

Deadman, P., Al-Khafaji, M. and Baker, K. (2001) *A Manual of Acupuncture*. Hove: Journal of Chinese Medicine Publications.

Deliaert, A.E., van den Elzen, M.E.P., van den Kerckhove, E., Fieuws, S. and van der Hulst, R.R.W.J. (2012) 'Smoking in Relation to Age in Aesthetic Facial Surgery.' *Aesthetic Plastic Surgery 36*, 4, 853–856.

Del Rosso, J.Q. and Levin, J. (2011) 'The Clinical Relevance of Maintaining the Functional Integrity of the Stratum Corneum in Both Healthy and Disease-Affected Skin.' *The Journal of Clinical and Aesthetic Dermatology 4*, 9, 22–42.

Eckman, P. (1996) *In the Footsteps of the Yellow Emperor*. San Francisco, CA: Cypress Book Company.

Emoto, M. (2004) *The Hidden Messages in Water*, trans. David A. Thayne. Hillsboro, OR: Beyond Hills Publishing.

Fabbrocini, G., Fardella, N., Monfrecola, A., Proietti, I. and Innocenzi, D. (2009) 'Acne Scarring Treatment Using Skin Needling.' *Clinical and Experimental Dermatology 34*, 8, 874–879.

Feng, C. and Zheng, C. (1994) 'Ancient Caves Reveal a Brilliant Medical World.' *American Journal of Chinese Medicine XXII*, 1, 95–99.

Frank, B. and Soliman, N. (1999) 'Zero Point: A Critical Assessment through Advanced Auricular Therapy.' *Medical Acupuncture 11*, 1, 13–16.

Goldberg, D.J. and Berlin, A. (2012) *Acne and Rosacea: Epidemiology, Diagnosis and Treatment*. London: Manson Publishing.

Gori, L. and Firenzuoli, F. (2007) 'Ear Acupuncture in European Traditional Medicine.' *Evidence-Based Complementary and Alternative Medicine 4*, 1, 13–16.

Hecker, H-U., Steveling, A., Peuker, E.T. and Kastner, J. (2005) *Practice of Acupuncture: Point Location, Treatment Options, TCM Basics*, trans. Ursula Vielkind. Stuttgart: Georg Thieme.

Herrmann, C.-M. (2000) *The Five Elements Volume I: The Movement of Life through Body, Mind and Spirit*. Coventry: Paul Coughlin.

Hicks, A. and Hicks, J. (1999) *Healing Your Emotions: Discover Your Element Type and Change Your Life*. London: Thorsons.

Jefferies, R. (2010) *The Life of the Fields*. New York, NY: Cambridge University Press.

Jiang, D., Liang, J. and Noble, P.W. (2007) 'Hyaluronan in Tissue Injury and Repair.' *Annual Review of Cell and Developmental Biology 23*, 435–461.

John, H.E. and Price, R.D. (2009) 'Perspectives in the Selection of Hyaluronic Acid Fillers for Facial Wrinkles and Aging Skin.' *Journal of Patient Preference and Adherence 3*, 225–230.

Kafi, R., Kwak, H.S.R., Schumacher, W.E., Cho, S. *et al.* (2007) 'Improvement of Naturally Aged Skin with Vitamin A (Retinol).' *Archives of Dermatology 143*, 5, 606–612.

Kahan, V., Anderson, M.L., Tomimori, J. and Tufik, S. (2010) 'Can Poor Sleep Affect Skin Integrity?' *Medical Hypotheses 75*, 6, 535–537.

Ken, C. and Yongqiang, C. (1991) *Handbook to Chinese Auricular Therapy*. Beijing: Foreign Languages Press.

Kidson, R.L. (2008) *Is Acupuncture Right for You? What It Is, Why It Works and How It Can Help You*. Rochester, VT: Healing Arts Press.

Larre, C. (1994) *The Way of Heaven, Neijing Suwen Chapters 1 and 2*, trans. P. Firebrace. Cambridge: Monkey Press.

Leung, L-H. (1997) 'A Stone that Kills Two Birds: How Pantothenic Acid Unveils the Mysteries of Acne Vulgaris and Obesity.' *Journal of Orthomolecular Medicine 12*, 2, 99–114.

Lushang, W. and Fei, X. (1997) 'Improving the Complexion by Needling Renying ST-9.' *Journal of Chinese Medicine 54*, 18–19.

Lyons, E. (1978) 'Chinese Jades – The Role of Jade in Ancient China: An Introduction to a Special Exhibition at the University Museum.' *Expedition 20*, 3, 4–20.

Mac-Mary, S., Sainthillier, J.-M., Jeudy, A., Sladen, C. *et al.* (2010) 'Assessment of Cumulative Exposure to UVA through the Study of Asymmetrical Facial Skin Aging.' *Clinical Interventions in Aging 5*, 277–284.

Majid, I. J. (2009) 'Microneedling Therapy in Atrophic Facial Scars: An Objective Assessment.' *Journal of Cutaneous and Aesthetic Surgery 2*, 1, 26–30.

Matsumoto, K. and Birch, S. (1986) *Extraordinary Vessels*. Brookline, MA: Paradigm Publications.

Meng, X., Xu, S. and Lao, L. (2011) 'Clinical Acupuncture Research in the West.' *Frontiers of Medicine 5*, 2, 134–140.

Nielsen, A. (1995) *Gua Sha: A Traditional Technique for Modern Practice*. Edinburgh: Churchill Livingstone.

Nielsen, A., Knoblauch, N.T.M., Dobos G.J., Michalsen, A. and Kaptchuk, T.J. (2007) 'The Effect of Gua Sha Treatment on the Microcirculation of Surface Tissue: A Pilot Study in Healthy Subjects.' *Explore 3*, 5, 456–466.

Papadimas, G.K., Tzirogiannis, K.N., Mykoniatis, M.G., Grypioti, A.D., Manta, G.A. and Panoutsopoulosm G.I. (2012) 'The Emerging Role of Serotonin in Liver Regeneration.' *Swiss Medical Weekly 142*, w13548, 1–6.

Pfab, F., Athanasiadis, G.I., Huss-Marp, J., FuQin, J. *et al.* (2011) 'Effect of Acupuncture on Allergen-Induced Basophil Activation in Patients with Atopic Eczema: A Pilot Trial.' *Journal of Alternative and Complementary Medicine 17*, 4, 309–314.

Reece, E.M., Pessa, J.E. and Rohrich, R.J. (2008) 'The Mandibular Septum: Anatomical Observations of the Jowls in Aging – Implications for Facial Rejuvenation.' *Plastic & Reconstructive Surgery 121*, 4, 1414–1420.

Reichstein, G. (1998) *Wood Becomes Water: Chinese Medicine in Everyday Life*. New York, NY: Kodansha America.

Reid, D. (2001) *Guarding the Three Treasures: The Chinese Way of Health*. London: Pocket Books.

Rochat de la Vallee, E. (2009) *Wu Xing: The Five Elements In Chinese Classical Texts*. Cambridge: Monkey Press.

Sharma, P., (2011) 'Cosmeceuticals: Regulatory Scenario in US, Europe and India.' *International Journal of Pharmacy & Technology 3*, 4, 1512–1535.

Sheikh, A. (2002) 'Itch, Sneeze and Wheeze: The Genetics of Atopic Dermatitis Allergy.' *Journal of the Royal Society of Medicine 95*, 1, 14–17.

Soulie de Morant, G. (1994) *Chinese Acupuncture*, trans. L. Grinnell, C. Jeanmougin and M. Leveque, ed. P. Zmiewski. Brookline, MA: Paradigm Publications.

Spoerel, W.E. (1975) 'Acupuncture Analgesia in China.' *American Journal of Chinese Medicine 3*, 4, 359–368.

Stener-Victorin, E., Waldenstrom, U., Nilsson, L., Wikland, M. and Janson, O.L. (1999) 'A Prospective Randomized Study of Electro-Acupuncture Versus Alfentanil as Anaesthesia during Oocyte Aspiration in In-vitro Fertilization.' *Human Reproduction 14*, 10, 2480–2484.

Sun, P., Li, L. and Si, M. (1992) 'Comparison of Acupuncture and Epidural Anesthesia in Appendectomy.' *Zhen Ci Yan Jiu 17*, 2, 87–89.

Tsu, Lao (1972) *Tao Te Ching*, trans. G.-F. Feng and J. English. New York, NY: Vintage Books.

Veith, I. (1972) *The Yellow Emperor's Classic of Internal Medicine*. Berkeley, CA: University of California Press.

Wallnofer, H. and Von Rottauscher, A. (1965) *Chinese Folk Medicine and Acupuncture*, trans. M. Palmedo. New York, NY: Bell Publishing Company.

Wang, H.-H., Chang, Y.H., Liu, D.-M. and Ho, Y.-J. (1997) 'A Clinical Study on Physiological Response in ElectroAcupuncture Anagesia and Meperidine Anagesia for Colonoscopy.' *American Journal of Chinese Medicine XXV*, 1, 13–20.

Wang, S.Y., Qu, X.X., Song, X.J., Li, S.Y., Ma, H.M. and Zhang, D. (2012) 'Blood Perfusion in Different Facial Acupoint Areas and Its Changes after Acupuncture Stimulation of Hegu (LI 4) Displayed by Laser Doppler Imager in Healthy Volunteers.' *Zhen Ci Yan Jiu 37*, 6, 482–487.

Wang, Y. and Oliver, G. (2010) 'Current Views on the Function of the Lymphatic Vasculature in Health and Disease.' *Genes and Development 24*, 2115–2126.

Whitman, W. (1888) 'The First Dandelion.' In *The Complete Poems of Walt Whitman* (1995). Ware: Wordsworth Editions.

Worsley, J.R. (1990) *Traditional Acupuncture Volume II: Traditional Diagnosis*. Leamington Spa: College of Traditional Acupuncture.

Worsley, J.R. (1998) *Classical Five-Element Acupuncture Volume III: The Five Elements and the Officials*. Gainsville, FL: Worsley Institute.

Xia, F., Han, J., Liu, X., Wang, J. *et al.* (2011) 'Prednisolone and Acupuncture in Bell's Palsy: Study Protocol for a Randomized, Controlled Trial.' *Trials 12*, 158.

Xu, S.-B., Huang, B., Zhang, C.-Y., Du, P. *et al.* (2013) 'Effectiveness of Strengthened Stimulation during Acupuncture for the Treatment of Bell Palsy: A Randomized Controlled Trial.' *Canadian Medical Association Journal 10*, 1503.

Yang, S.-Z. (1998) *The Divine Farmer's Materia Medica: A Translation of the Shen Nong Ben Cao Jing*. Boulder, CO: Blue Poppy Press.

Yang, S.-Z. and Chace, C. (1994) *The Systematic Classic of Acupuncture and Moxibustion by Huang Fu-Mi: A Translation of the Jia Yi Jing*. Boulder, CO: Blue Poppy Press.

Yang, Y., Ji, L., Li, G., Deng, X., Cai, P. and Guan, L. (2012) 'Differences in Thermal Effects of Moxibustion at Zusanli (ST 36) and Hegu (LI 4) on Various Facial Areas in Healthy People.' *Journal of Traditional Chinese Medicine 32*, 3, 397–403.

Zara, L. (2001) *Jade*. Lincoln, NE: iUniverse.com.

Zhang, P. (2006) *A Comprehensive Handbook for Traditional Chinese Medicine Facial Rejuvenation*. New York, NY: Nefeli Corporation.